Donor Organ Transplants or Blind for the football

AN UPLIFTING TALE OF DETERMINATION, PERSISTENCE, TENACITY & POSITIVITY

BILLY RYLE

Donor Organ Transplants or Blind for the football
By Billy Ryle

This book was first published in Great Britain in paperback during July 2023.

The moral right of Billy Ryle is to be identified as the author of this work and has been asserted by him in accordance with the Copyright, Designs and Patents Act of 1988.

All rights are reserved and no part of this book may be produced or utilized in any format, or by any means, electronic or mechanical, including photocopying, recording or by any information storage or retrieval system, without prior permission in writing from the publishers - Coast & Country/Ads2life. ads2life@btinternet.com

All rights reserved.

ISBN: 979-8851163746

Contents

Synopsis..i

The Author..ii

DEDICATION..iii

ACKNOWLEDGEMENTS..iv

CHILDREN'S RHYME FROM TIMES PAST v

ON HIS BLINDNESS vi

DIAGRAM: EYE ANATOMY vii

CHAPTER ONE DEVELOPING CATARACTS 1

CHAPTER TWO THE CATARACT BUS 5

CHAPTER THREE FUCHS DYSTROPHY..16

CHAPTER FOUR CATARACT SURGERY 23

CHAPTER FIVE MONITORING MY VISION......................................26

CHAPTER SIX CAMPAIGN FOR DIVING BOARDS 36

CHAPTER SEVEN THE BENEFITS OF SEA SWIMMING.................47

CHAPTER EIGHT THE NOVEL..50

CHAPTER NINE NEW CONSULTANT OPHTHALMIC SURGEON 60

CHAPTER TEN RIGHT EYE CATARACT SURGERY 65

CHAPTER ELEVEN MISTER CHAIRMAN 73

CHAPTER TWELVE CATARACT SURGERY SUCCESS 80

CHAPTER THIRTEEN BUSY DIARY 84

CHAPTER FOURTEEN ROCK & ROSE VICTORY SOCIAL..............92

CHAPTER FIFTEEN LOCKDOWN...120

CHAPTER SIXTEEN A COVID FUNERAL..124

CHAPTER SEVENTEEN THE BRACKER 100KM WALK 132

CHAPTER EIGHTEEN CLUB TITLE BUT CHAMPIONSHIP EXIT.......148

CHAPTER NINETEEN WALK THE WALK..154

CHAPTER TWENTY 1920 COMMEMORATION CEREMONY 158

CHAPTER TWENTY ONE CONSIDERING A CORNEAL TRANSPLANT 166

CHAPTER TWENTY TWO UNDERSTANDING CORNEAL SURGERY 170

CHAPTER TWENTY THREE PUBLIC HEALTH GUIDELINES 174

CHAPTER TWENTY FOUR FOCUS ON SENIOR COUNTY CHAMPIONSHIP...179

CHAPTER TWENTY FIVE GAA DISCIPLINE...185

CHAPTER TWENTY SIX DETERIORATING VISION 188

CHAPTER TWENTY SEVEN GOOD MENTAL HEALTH 191

CHAPTER TWENTY EIGHT A NOD & A WINK TO ANTHONY DALY 195

CHAPTER TWENTY NINE ONE GOOD ADULT TO LISTEN 201

CHAPTER THIRTY DISABILITY PATH 208

CHAPTER THIRTY ONE PROMOTION FOR SENIOR B TEAM 216

CHAPTER THIRTY TWO THREE IN A ROW SENIOR CLUB CHAMPIONS 222

CHAPTER THIRTY THREE A DATE FOR CORNEAL TRANSPLANTATION 228

CHAPTER THIRTY FOUR PROGRESS IN COUNTY SENIOR CHAMPIONSHIP...231

CHAPTER THIRTY FIVE PENALTY SHOOT OUT IN SEMI-FINAL 236

CHAPTER THIRTY SIX KERRY SENIOR FOOTBALL CHAMPIONS ..245

CHAPTER THIRTY SEVEN PSYCHOLOGICAL WARFARE 259

CHAPTER THIRTY EIGHT NEW DATE FOR SURGERY 265

CHAPTER THIRTY NINE THE DREAM DIES IN THURLES 271

CHAPTER FORTY STEPPING DOWN..278

CHAPTER FORTY ONE ANOTHER SETBACK 286

CHAPTER FORTY TWO FIRST CORNEAL TRANSPLANT 289

CHAPTER FORTY THREE AFTERCARE OF NEW CORNEA...............294

CHAPTER FORTY FOUR CATARACT & CORNEA 297

CHAPTER FORTY FIVE ENJOYING THE GAMES................................. 300

CHAPTER FORTY SIX COMBINED SURGERY...................................... 303

CHAPTER FORTY SEVEN CHALAZION 307

CHAPTER FORTY EIGHT THE CHARGE TO THE SEA 310

CHAPTER FORTY NINE OUTPATIENT... 313

CHAPTER FIFTY HELEN KELLER & ANNE SULLIVAN.................... 316

CHAPTER FIFTY ONE RAFTERY THE POET 321

CHAPTER FIFTY TWO THE BLIND SINGERS 327

CHAPTER FIFTY THREE VISUALLY IMPAIRED IRISH
PERSONALITIES 338

CHAPTER FIFTY FOUR NATIONAL COUNCIL FOR THE BLIND OF
IRELAND.. 351

CHAPTER FIFTY FIVE IRISH GUIDE DOGS FOR THE BLIND............ 358

CHAPTER FIFTY SIX INEQUALITY, DISABILITY & KINDNESS 363

Synopsis

Billy Ryle was enjoying a full and active life. He was blessed with good health, enjoyed his job and loved outdoor living and sport. Like his parents before him, the time came for him to need reading glasses. He then graduated to wearing glasses fulltime for reading and distance sight.

On a routine visit to Dr Tom O'Regan, Ophthalmologist to have his eyes examined, he was informed that he had cataracts developing in both eyes and was referred to Mr David Wallace, Consultant Ophthalmologist, Bon Secours Hospital, Tralee, whose diagnosis of Fuchs Dystrophy was totally unexpected and alarming. In Fuchs Dystrophy, fluid builds up in the clear layer (cornea) on the front of the eye, causing the cornea to swell and thicken. This leads to glare, blurred or cloudy vision, and eye discomfort. Fuchs Dystrophy usually affects both eyes, causing the vision to gradually worsen leading to blindness.

It was the beginning of a difficult medical journey, involving two cataract surgeries and two corneal transplant operations of donor organs at Bon Secours Hospital, Cork by Mr Tom Flynn, Consultant Ophthalmic Surgeon, which Billy was determined to make in order to save his sight.

Simultaneously, as Chairman of Austin Stacks GAA Club, Tralee he was determined to lead his Club safely through the Covid-19 pandemic to win the Kerry Senior Football Championship in 2021. Billy tells his story in this engrossing narrative.

The Author

Billy Ryle, Career Guidance Counsellor, author and freelance writer is an avid reader who contributes regularly to a number of newspapers, pamphlets and magazines. He has a long-standing interest in career and educational counselling.

Billy's first book was, 'Second Level Study Guide - A Plan for Exam Success,' directed at second level students who were preparing for the State Examinations in Ireland. His second book, 'From Fenit Bathing Slip to the High Court – a five -year journey of honour' was published in May 2017.

Billy's first novel 'Christian Brotherly Love' was published in 2019. He was also a major contributor to and editorial team member of 'A Centenary History, 1917-2017, Austin Stacks GAA Club Tralee Co. Kerry,' which was published in December 2017.

Billy attended Mercy Primary School Tralee, Co. Kerry, CBS Primary & Secondary Schools, Tralee, Co. Kerry. He studied at University College Cork for a BA, HDE and Diploma in Career Guidance. He also holds a Master of Education Degree from University of Galway.

Billy has enjoyed a lifetime of active involvement in sport, community development and voluntary work. He won numerous awards as player and coach at swimming, basketball, Gaelic football and hurling. He is an active member, former Chairman and Secretary of Austin Stack's GAA Club, Tralee and enjoys history, crosswords, humour, table quiz and mathematics. Billy is an all-year-round swimmer at the bathing slip in Fenit, Tralee, Co. Kerry. He is a practising and progressive Catholic.

Billy lives with his wife, Sheila in Spa, Tralee, Co. Kerry. They have three adult children, Kevin, a General Medical Practitioner, Gráinne, a Pharmacist and Brian, a Dental Surgeon.

DEDICATION

To

Mr Tom Flynn, Consultant Ophthalmic Surgeon

&

Dr Tom O'Regan, Ophthalmologist

With my thanks & gratitude

Net profit from the sale of this Book during 2023 will be donated to the National Council for the Blind of Ireland (NCBI)

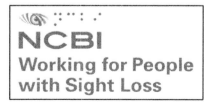

ACKNOWLEDGEMENTS

Adrienne McLoughlin, Photography

American Association of the Deaf-Blind

Anne Sullivan Foundation for people who are Deafblind

Carol Anne O Donoghue, Photography

David Wallace, Consultant Ophthalmologist, Notes on the Eye

Dermot Crean, Tralee Today, Photography

Focus on Diversity

Guide Dogs of Hawaii

Helen Keller Foundation- Seeing the Possibilities

Irish Examiner Newspaper

Irish Guide Dogs for the Blind

John Cleary, Photography

Jim Naughton, former Chairman, Austin Stacks GAA Club, Tralee

Kerry's Eye Newspaper

Mairéad Fernane, former Chairperson, Austin Stacks GAA Club, Tralee

Martin Cleary, Photography

Martin Collins, PRO, Austin Stacks GAA Club, Tralee

Michael Carroll, Austin Stacks GAA Club, Tralee

National Council for the Blind of Ireland (NCBI)

Paddy Barry, Team Manager, Austin Stacks GAA Club, Tralee

Shane Lynch, Chairman, Austin Stacks GAA Club, Tralee

Tom Flynn, Consultant Ophthalmic Surgeon, Notes on the Eye

The Kerryman Newspaper

Tralee Today Online News

Wikipedia

CHILDREN'S RHYME FROM TIMES PAST

"I see" said the blind man "a hole in the wall"

"You fool" said the deaf man "you can't see at all"

"You're the fool" said the mute man "you can't hear at all"

THE BLIND MAN CAN'T SEE, THE DEAF MAN CAN'T HEAR AND THE MUTE MAN CAN'T SPEAK. PERHAPS THE RHYME IS REMINDING EACH OF US TO BE AWARE OF OUR OWN DISABILITIES AND TO BE SENSITIVE TO THE DISABILITIES OF OTHERS!

ON HIS BLINDNESS

by
JOHN MILTON

When I consider how my light is spent

Ere half my days in this dark world and wide,

And that one talent which is death to hide

Lodged with me useless, though my soul more bent

To serve therewith my Maker, and present

My true account, lest he returning chide,

"Doth God exact day-labour, light denied?"

I fondly ask. But Patience, to prevent

That murmur, soon replies: "God doth not need

Either man's work or his own gifts: who best

Bear his mild yoke, they serve him best. His state

Is kingly; thousands at his bidding speed

And post o'er land and ocean without rest:

They also serve who only stand and wait.

The famous sonnet was written by English poet John Milton around 1650 as he was losing his sight. Milton was completely blind by 1652 at 43yrs of age. In the poem, Milton reflects on the tragedy and frustration of his visual impairment and his fear that he won't be able to serve God without his sight. Eventually Milton realises that by accepting his blindness he will continue to serve God.

EYE ANATOMY

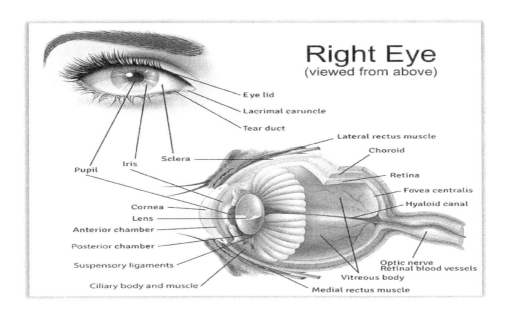

The seven parts of the eye

Sclera: The white protective outer layer of the eye.

Cornea: The transparent front segment of the eye that covers the iris, pupil and anterior chamber, and provides most of the eye's optical power.

Iris: Coloured tissue lying behind the cornea that gives colour to the eye (e.g., blue eyes, brown eyes) and controls the amount of light entering the eye by varying size of the black pupillary opening.

Pupil: A black circular opening in the centre of the iris that regulates the amount of light that enters the eye.

Lens: Transparent, intraocular tissue that helps bring rays of light to focus on the retina. A cataract is a lens that has become cloudy or opaque.

Retina: The part of the eye that converts images from the eye's optical system into electrical impulses sent along the optic nerve for transmission to the brain. The retina lines the rear two-thirds of the eye and consists of layers that include rods and cones. This part of the eye can be compared to film in a camera.

Optic Nerve: The primary sensory nerve of the eye. It carries impulses for sight from the retina to the brain.

CHAPTER ONE

DEVELOPING CATARACTS

As the saying goes, health is wealth. It's a saying I never gave too much thought to until I made an appointment for a routine eye check in late 2017. I had been wearing glasses for a considerable number of years, beginning with reading glasses and then progressing on to wearing glasses full time for reading and long-distance vision. I put the need for glasses down to the normal aging process and to my genetic inheritance from my parents. My father wore glasses fulltime and my mother wore reading glasses. In addition, as an avid reader, I became more dependent on glasses to read books with varying font sizes.

My appointment with Dr Tom O'Regan, Ophthalmologist was primarily to establish if I needed to switch to glasses with stronger lenses as I had recently noticed a deterioration in the clarity of my current bifocals. I expected nothing more than a thorough check on the quality of my vision and a new prescription for glasses which would improve my vision. What a shock I got when Dr O'Regan informed me that I had cataracts developing in both eyes. The Doctor informed me that, in the not-to-distant future, I would need surgery in both eyes to have the cataracts removed.

I knew little or nothing about cataracts other than what I regularly heard on radio and television. I knew it was a condition that affected the vision of a considerable number of people as they grew older. Apparently, there was a long waiting list for cataract surgery in the public health service and a number of politicians were arranging transport for people to travel to Belfast where corrective surgery was more readily available for those who could pay on the day. A refund of the cost of the operation would subsequently be made by the Government on submission of receipts. I also learned that the operation was available, with little or no delay, in private hospitals in the Republic of Ireland, to those who had health insurance or the means to pay for the procedure.

This was the first time I gave any serious thought to the two-tier health system that exists in the Republic of Ireland. A person who was dependent on the public hospital system had a long wait for all but emergency health care, while someone like myself with health insurance could avail of the private hospital system. The more I thought about it the more unfair the two-tier system seemed to me. I discussed the matter with my family – my wife and my three children are all health care professionals – to be told that I had a valid concern but there was little or nothing I could do to correct or improve the health care system. In fact, by going private rather than public, I wouldn't be adding to an already lengthy list of people languishing on the public hospital waiting list.

So, in order to prepare for the appointment which Dr O'Regan was arranging for me with Mr David Wallace, Consultant Ophthalmologist at the Bon Secours Hospital, Tralee, I decided to find out as much as I could about a cataract. I began by looking at a diagram of the eye. The cornea is a window of transparent tissue at the front of the eyeball, which allows light to pass into the eye and provides focus so that images can be seen. The iris is the circular-coloured part inside the eye. The little black hole in the middle of the iris is called the pupil. The lens is directly behind the iris and pupil. In a normal eye, the lens is clear. It helps to focus light rays on to the retina at the back of the eye. This sends messages to the brain to allow us see. A cataract is clouding of the lens. When cataract develops, the lens becomes cloudy and prevents the light rays from passing through.

Apparently, cataracts form slowly over the years and gradually cause a blurring of the vision, which cannot be corrected by wearing glasses. In some people, the quality of vision deteriorates very quickly. A developing cataract can also cause glare, difficulty with night driving and multiple images in one eye can affect the quality of one's vision. Cataracts don't spread from eye to eye, but they often develop in both eyes at the same time or one after the other with a time interval in between. Most forms of cataract develop in later life. This is called age-related cataract and can occur any time after the age of forty years. The normal process of aging causes the lens to gradually become cloudy. Not every person who develops cataract requires treatment. Apparently, there is no known method of preventing cataract.

In many cases cataract is harmless and can be left in one's eye. It is usually safe not to have surgery if one feels that there is no problem with one's vision or if one does not wish to have an operation. But, when the cataract progresses to the point where it is interfering with daily activities or lifestyle, even when using up-to-date glasses, then cataract surgery may be the best course of action.

Modern surgery is highly successful for the majority of patients but, as is the case with all surgery, there are risks. Cataract surgery is performed when one has a problem with vision and wants to do something about it.

It is very common for a cataract to develop in one eye more quickly than in the other. The timing of an operation is agreed after discussion between the Doctor and the patient. Usually, the more seriously affected eye is operated on first. Sometimes, it's advisable to have the second eye operated on, even if it's causing few vision symptoms, in order that both eyes can be comfortably used together.

While it is possible to operate on both eyes together this is not routinely done. Simultaneous bilateral – both eyes at the same time – cataract surgery is only performed on a specific needs-basis. The Doctor in charge of the patient's treatment is the best person to advise on the suitability, as well as the risks and benefits, of having surgery on both eyes at the same time.

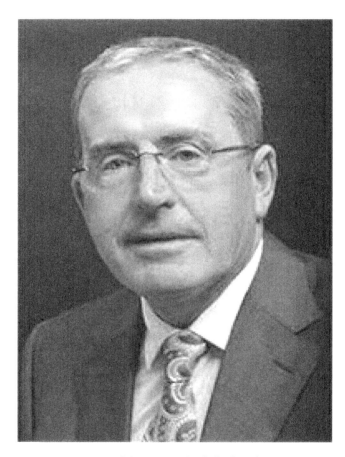

Dr Tom O'Regan, Ophthalmologist

CHAPTER TWO

THE CATARACT BUS

I have been a lifelong active member of my local GAA Club, Austin Stacks, The Rock, Tralee, which celebrated its centenary year in 2017. As part of the celebration of the club's one hundred years in existence, a committee of members, who were known to have an interest in writing, was set up to research the history of the club from 1917 and to present it in book format towards the end of 2017. In addition to myself, the other members of the group were Martin Collins, Tadgh McMahon, Eddie Barrett, Kerry O'Shea, Tony O'Keeffe, Tim Slattery, Adrienne McLoughlin and Seamus Smith. It was a pleasure to be a member of such a very dedicated team and I really enjoyed working on the project, which took the best part of two years. The book, which we named 'A Centenary History, 1917 – 2017, Austin Stacks GAA Club, The Rock, Tralee, Co. Kerry,' was launched by our Club Chairman, Liam Lynch at our facilities in Connolly Park, Tralee on Friday, 15th December, 2017.

In retrospect, the research, the interviews, the long hours and late nights spent on reading, editing, correcting, rewriting, sourcing photographs and all of the other aspects which are part and parcel of producing a major publication, may not have done my eyes any favours but the beautiful end product made it all worthwhile. I felt very proud to have been a member of a committee which documented the wonderful story of a club for which I have a great affection and which I carry in my heart wherever I travel.

I was also given the honour of speaking at the launch on behalf of the book committee. Our club house was packed to capacity and there was a great atmosphere as everybody present was very keen to buy a copy of the book. Having learned a few days earlier from Dr O' Regan that cataracts were developing in my eyes, my confidence in my vision was beginning to flag, so I made sure to print my speech in an extra-large font. In the event, my few words were well received and I had nothing to worry about. My speech, which I have reduced to standard font for inclusion in this book, is published below. A section of the speech was delivered in Irish, but, for the convenience of readers, I have presented it below entirely in English.

I began by welcoming Brendan Dowling, President of Austin Stacks, Liam Lynch, Chairman of Austin Stacks, club members, club supporters, special guests and friends to that very special occasion. I pointed out that we were gathered at our clubhouse in Connolly Park where our centenary book, containing the one-hundred-year history of our beloved club was being launched by our Chairman, Liam Lynch. I mentioned that the members of the centenary book committee - Martin Collins, Tadgh Mc Mahon, Eddie Barrett, Kerry O Shea, Tony O Keeffe, Tim Slattery, Adrienne McLoughlin, Seamus Smith and myself were delighted that this beautiful book was being launched on that particular evening.

"Almost two years ago," I said, "Liam invited a group of us to research and to write the centenary book. We held our first meeting on 11th March 2016 and we have worked tirelessly ever since to produce a history to do justice to one hundred years of the Rock Club. In that objective we have succeeded with aplomb. Tonight, we are proud to present a beautiful book of aesthetic appeal, superb photography and a captivating narrative from beginning to end.

All seven of us on the editorial team brought a variety of skills to the table but I know my colleagues will agree that Martin Collins and Tadgh McMahon provided the leadership, the energy, the determination and the passion to get this project over the line. Martin and Tadgh have worked selflessly and altruistically to deliver this book, expecting nothing in return, other than the satisfaction of accurately recording a centenary story. They are two exceptional Rockies and they epitomize all that is good and wholesome about this wonderful club.

The energetic Séamus Smith was our information technology expert for the duration. He introduced us to the digital world of drop boxes and cloud computing and he played a huge part in preparing the book for printing.

The courteous Adrienne McLoughlin made a huge contribution to this book. She shot the entire range of contemporary photographs in her relaxed and unflappable style. Her beautiful work permeates this book from cover to cover. The Rock is very fortunate to have the photographic talent of Adrienne at its disposal.

A great deal of the book was written by the seven-member editorial team. To give you a little flavour - Tony sets the scene in a unique and well researched preface. Tim provides a century of facts and figures. Kerry has the heroes of our first golden era jumping off the page. Eddie delivers an excellent profile of Austin Stack and an array of past years' photographs. You'll come across all of this and much more as you read the book, but I'd also like to acknowledge outstanding contributions from a number of guest writers.

Big Dan written by his niece and Club Vice-Chairperson, Mairéad Fernane
Rory written by the late great Paddy Drummond and published by kind permission of the Drummond/McMahon families
Juvenile articles by Mícheál Hayes (The Master) and Colm Mangan
Mná na Carraige by Ann O Callaghan Eager and Noreen Power
Past Memories by Jo Jo Barrett
Hurling by John Barry, Ger Scollard and Brian Neenan
Cultural Activities by Brian Caball
Purty written by Matt Leen
The Future by Liam Lynch

Our sincere thanks must also go to Aogán Ó Fearghail, President, Gaelic Athletic Association, Diarmuid Ó Súilleabháin, Chairman, Munster GAA Council and Liam O Loinsigh, Chairman, Austin Stacks GAA Club, who wrote the introduction at the beginning of the book.

I'd like to fondly mention Mick Ryan, who did a lovely interview with us last year and Denis O Connor who provided us with a meeting venue at any time of day or night. The final whistle blew for those loyal Rockies before the book was published.

The nine of us on the book committee would like to dedicate the very first copy off the printing press to all the deceased, who played any part in the club during its first centenary. I sense their presence all around us here tonight. This book guarantees that they will never be forgotten. It's my pleasure to present Liam with this first copy, which has been signed by all of its contributors."

After the formalities of that very special launch, we all enjoyed refreshments courtesy of our very active ladies' committee. Many people approached myself and my fellow authors, to congratulate us on our achievement and to say how much they were looking forward to reading the book and looking through the fabulous array of photographs that were featured in the book. One of those who approached me, was an acquaintance whom I hadn't seen for some time.

"Well, hello stranger, long time no see," I jokingly remarked.

"Congrats on a great publication, which, I'm sure, will read as well as it looks," my fellow club member replied. "I wasn't able to attend many matches during the past year as I had some trouble with my eyes."

He had my immediate and undivided attention and I was determined to listen to his story. He told me that he had noticed a deterioration in his eye sight at the beginning of the year. He described it as a blur or haze in his vision which he thought would pass in time. He had never worn glasses at this stage but as the condition was affecting the quality of his life, he eventually decided the time had come to make an appointment with an Optician. Similar to myself, he rarely missed a football match in which Austin Stacks was involved but was finding it increasingly more difficult to recognise the players and to follow the play. The Optician confirmed that he needed cataract surgery.

Unfortunately, he didn't have private health insurance and when he enquired, he was told that there was a considerable waiting list for cataract surgery in the public health system. Fortunately, he had some savings put aside for a rainy day so he was able to travel to Belfast on the 'Cataract Bus,' where he had a very successful operation in his right eye. Most of his costs were repaid in due course by the Health Service Executive and he was finalising arrangements to return to Belfast in the new year to have the same procedure carried out on his left eye.

'If I hadn't the few euro in the Bank, Billy boy, it could have been years before I would again watch a match but within a few months I expect to be back on the terrace supporting The Rockies,' he said.

When I thought about it later, I felt a deep sense of gratitude to the Association of Secondary Teachers in Ireland (ASTI), the secondary teachers' union which I had joined at the beginning of my teaching career. The ASTI had set up a private health insurance group scheme with the VHI for all of its members and their families. Not only had the ASTI negotiated a competitive price for group membership but it had also arranged for the payments to be deducted directly in instalments from members' salary after the relevant income tax relief had been applied. We teachers had lifelong private health insurance for ourselves and our families without the worry of having to come up with a one off expensive annual payment.

Another huge service provided by the ASTI for its members was the superannuation scheme which guaranteed each retiring teacher a gratuity and a decent pension. The value of that scheme became crystal clear to me when I retired from my career as a secondary teacher a few years ago.

The ASTI is an outstanding trade union which works tirelessly on behalf of its members. I was very happy to give something back to my trade union as a school steward, as a delegate to Annual Conference, as Vice Chairman of the Kerry Branch and as ASTI National Convenor for Guidance and Counselling.

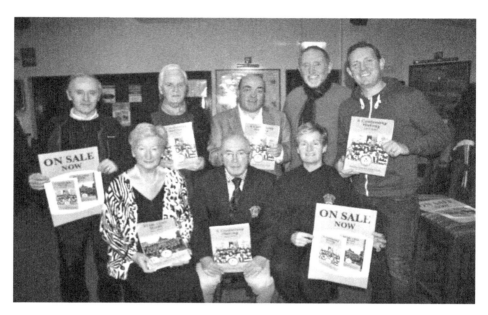

At the Press Conference on 11th December 2017 to announce the launch of Austin Stacks Centenary History Book were Front L/R: Mairéad Fernane, Vice-Chairperson, Martin Collins and Adrienne McLoughlin Back L/r: Tim Slattery, Tadgh McMahon, Kerry O'Shea, Billy Ryle and Stephen Smith

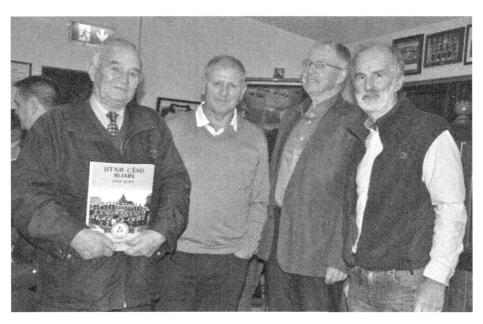

At the launch of Austin Stacks Centenary History Book on 15th December 2017 were L/r: Micheál Hayes, Ger McNamara, Colm Mangan and Fergus Dillon

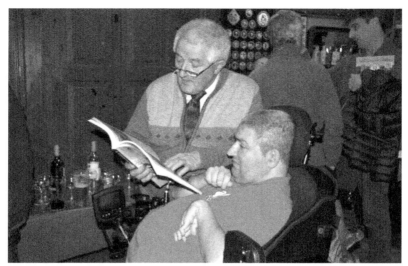

At the launch of Austin Stacks Centenary History Book on 15th December 2017 were George Dineen Snr and George Dineen

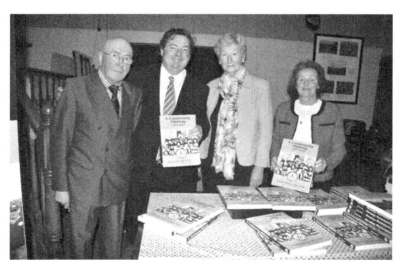

At the launch of Austin Stacks Centenary History Book on 15th December 2017 were L/r: Martin Collins, Eddie Barrett, Mairéad Fernane and Carmel Quilter O'Neill

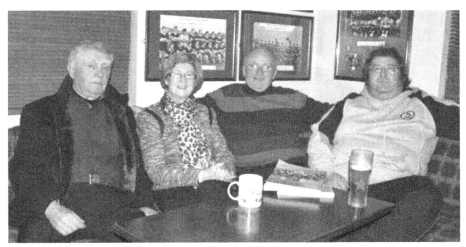

At the launch of Austin Stacks Centenary History Book on 15th December 2017 were L/r: Brendan Dowling, Club President, Eileen & Séamus McCarthy and Ger Scollard

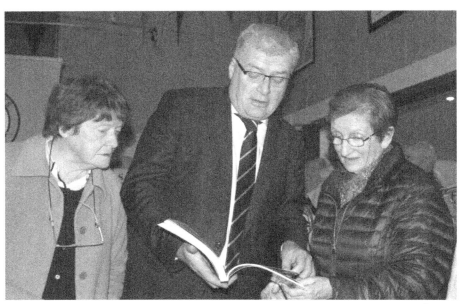

At the launch of Austin Stacks Centenary History Book on 15th December 2017 were L/r: Phil Lynch, Liam Lynch, Club Chairman and Nuala Ryan

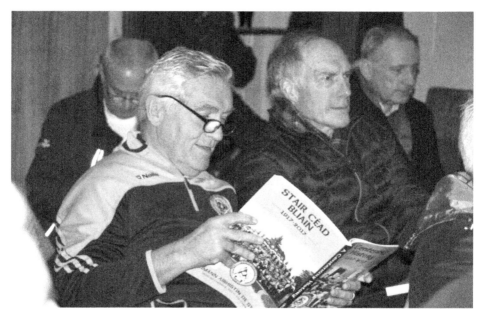

At the launch of Austin Stacks Centenary History Book on 15th December 2017 were Ger Power, left, and John O'Keeffe

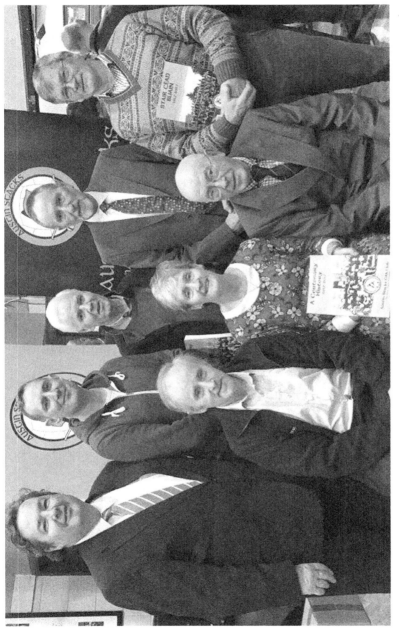

The "Book Committee" pictured at the launch of Austin Stacks Centenary History Book on 15th December 2017 were Front L/r: Tim Slattery, Adrienne McLoughlin and Martin Collins. Back L/r: Eddie Barrett, Stephen Smith, Tadgh Mc Mahon, Billy Ryle and Tony O'Keeffe. Absent from picture is Kerry O'Shea

CHAPTER THREE

FUCHS DYSTROPHY

In early January 2018, I attended an appointment which Dr. O'Regan had arranged for me with Mr David Wallace, Consultant Ophthalmologist, Bon Secours Hospital, Tralee. My eyes were given a very thorough examination by Mr Wallace who shocked me by telling me that not only was there evidence of bilateral early cataracts but that slit lamp microscopy revealed Fuchs Endothelial Dystrophy. My situation was far more serious than I had expected. On my way into Mr Wallace, I had accepted that, in the not-too-distant future it would be necessary for me to have cataract surgery in one eye, followed by a similar procedure in the second eye sometime later. To be informed that I had Fuchs Dystrophy was another matter altogether. The name of the disease, in itself, frightened the life out of me. Here I was living the good life, reading books, writing articles, having a daily sea swim, enjoying the football matches without a care in the world. It looked as if my world, at least my visual world, was about to come tumbling down.

Dr Wallace reassured me by informing me that medical intervention was available for both cataracts and Fuchs Dystrophy, which would require a corneal transplant in each eye. The mention of 'transplant' left me in no doubt that I that I had a serious battle ahead of me in the next few years. I recalled reading about a transplant for the first time when Dr Christiaan Barnard, a South African Cardiac Surgeon performed the first human-to-human heart transplant operation on the 3rd December 1967. It was a pioneering procedure which captured the imagination of the world. I'm not sure if it was the first time that an organ from one person was transplanted in the body of another person, but it certainly made Dr Bernard famous world-wide and brought hope to those who needed an organ transplant. I have been aware since of people receiving transplants of other organs such as liver, kidney and lung.

Indeed, I was very impressed by the altruistic gesture by Joe Brolly, former Derry footballer, Belfast based Barrister and GAA analyst in donating one of his kidneys to a club colleague a few years ago. Joe is a man who shoots from the hip in his commentary and he is a controversial figure in GAA circles with his no-holds barred views on Gaelic football. However, he showed tremendous courage and empathy by donating a kidney to Shane Finnegan, his colleague in St. Brigid's GAA Club, Belfast. Joe Brolly said that he was honoured to have been in a position to help Shane, who had been waiting for a transplant for over six years.

"He's been waiting for a transplant for over six years and when I heard that the only possibility of one was through a live donor I contacted his medical team," Brolly said.

Joe Brolly's donation of a kidney to Shane Finnegan was a selfless and compassionate act of friendship, which very few people would be brave enough to emulate. I carry an organ donor card in my wallet, which states that I wish to donate my kidneys, eyes, heart, lungs and liver to help others after my death. Fair enough, but would I have the bottle to do what Joe Brolly did? Probably not, unless it was a last resort. My organs are freely available after my death but until that happens, I'd prefer to leave them where they are.

Joe Brolly, of course, is fondly remembered in my own Austin Stacks GAA Club as the anti-hero, who was put in his place by our adored star man, Kieran Donaghy. Brolly had more or less written off any chances of Kerry doing well in the 2014 All-Ireland series. Kieran went on to play a starring role in Kerry's 2-09 to 0-12 All-Ireland final triumph over Donegal and in the immediate aftermath of that victory, he reserved special mention for the Sunday Game analyst when he looked directly at the RTE camera in Croke Park and said in an animated voice:

"I think Joe Brolly told us the production line was finished in Kerry - well, Joe Brolly, what do you think of that?"

The following January, about four months after posing the question live on air, Kieran Donaghy finally found out in person what Joe Brolly thought of Kerry when the outspoken Gaelic football pundit made a surprise appearance at an Austin Stacks fundraiser. Brolly was flown in from Belfast for Austin Stack's corporate lunch in Ballygarry House Hotel, Tralee in aid of the Club's new pitch purchase and development. Donaghy was on stage with compere Eoin McDevitt when Brolly came through the doors after the Kerry captain's now famous post-final speech was replayed on close circuit TVs for the attendance. Donaghy joked that Brolly was the one pundit to whom he gave some credibility but when the Derry man questioned his future on the Kerry team, it had an effect on him.

Brolly replied: "I'll tell you something. It wasn't me who left you on the bench for five or six games of the season."

Asked by McDevitt if he wanted to apologise to Donaghy, Brolly responded: "Are you serious? I got this man an All Star!"

Donaghy fired back: "We both didn't do too bad out of it, Joe!"

By all accounts, Kieran and Joe have remained firm friends ever since.

Organ donation got a huge fillip, a few years ago, in my home town of Tralee, when a tree was planted in the beautiful town park as a memorial to organ donors. In May, 2014, Councillor Mairéad Fernane of Tralee Town Council put forward a motion that a tree be planted, dedicated to organ donors, in acknowledgement of the huge contribution that they make to the lives of others. Mairéad told her fellow councillors that the tree would help to raise awareness of the importance of organ donation. It would provide people, whose late loved ones had donated organs or who had benefitted from organ donations, with a special place to visit, to think, to reflect and to pay their respects. Mairéad's thoughtful motion got the full and enthusiastic support of her fellow councillors and managerial staff.

Since I myself became the beneficiary of organ donations of two different decedents, the tree has added significance for me. The ornamental Japanese Flowering Cherry tree, Prunus Serrulata in Latin, is thriving in an area of scenic beauty in the town park. Against the background of a colourful arrangement of flowers, shrubs and trees, one can take a few moments away from the hustle and bustle of daily living to offer up a silent prayer for those who were generous enough to give others the gift of life or to occasion a huge improvement in the quality of their lives. Organ donors, such as Joe Brolly, are philanthropic and special people. Many of them, including my own donors remain anonymous, but this beautiful deciduous tree that produces a bountiful harvest of beautiful pinkish-red blossoms each spring in Tralee's town park means that organ donors will always be fondly remembered.

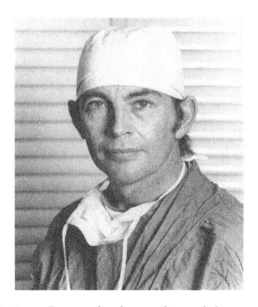

Dr Christiaan Barnard, who performed the world's first heart transplant operation in 1967

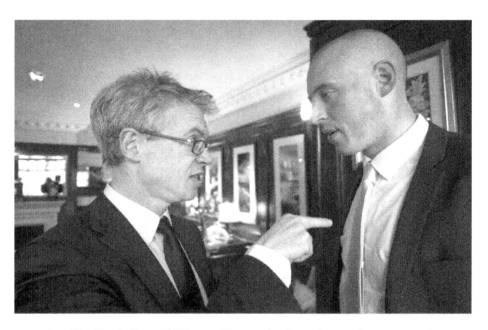

Joe Brolly, left, and Kieran Donaghy in animated conversation

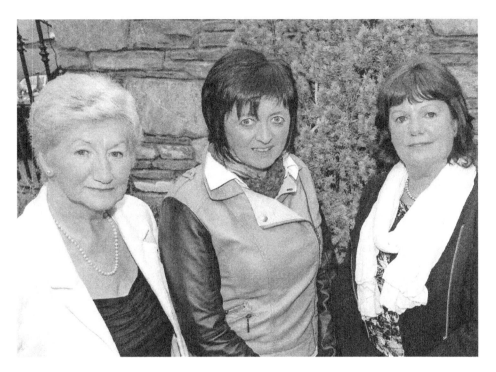

Pictured at a special meeting to recognise Organ Transplant week at Meadowlands Hotel, Tralee on Wednesday, 9th April, 2014 are
L/r- Councillor Mairéad Fernane, Meeting Organiser & Chairperson, Teresa Looney, Chairperson of the Kerry Irish Kidney Association and Phyllis Cunningham, National Transplant Co-Ordinator, Beaumont Hospital, Dublin

Photo Courtesy of Kerry's Eye

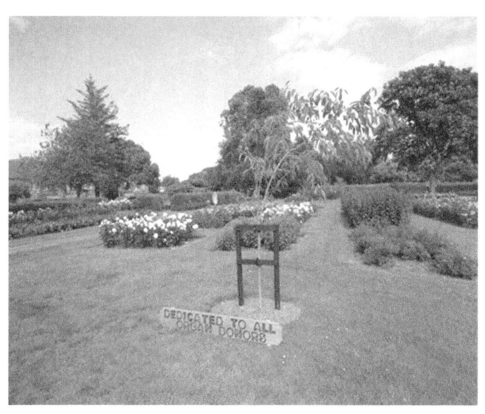

The tree in the town park, Tralee, Co. Kerry which is dedicated to all organ donors

CHAPTER FOUR

CATARACT SURGERY

As I mentioned earlier, subsequent to my appointment with Dr O'Regan, I did some reading about cataracts, but Mr Wallace gave me a great understanding of the condition and the required surgery. I studied, in some detail and repeatedly, the very reader friendly literature which he provided me with. The literature defined what a cataract actually is, what causes it, when to have surgery and what happens on the day of surgery. It was very reassuring literature for a person without a medical background and was a great preparation for what lay ahead.

What is a cataract?
 It's a cloudiness of the lens of the eye. Normally the lens is transparent and used to focus light onto the back of the eye, called 'the retina.' That allows a person to see things clearly. If a cataract develops the vision becomes reduced. Depending on the degree of cloudiness of the lens, a cataract can cause visual symptoms ranging from mild haziness to almost total blindness. As a cataract develops, so does the blurring and a point is reached where a change of glasses won't improve vision. When that stage is reached, the only effective treatment is surgery.

What causes cataract?
Most cataracts are caused by changes in the lens as a person ages. It can also be caused by inflammation in the eye, certain drugs and other medical conditions such as diabetes.

When should a person have surgery?
A cataract doesn't have to be removed because it is in the eye. It doesn't do anything other than impair a person's vision in the particular eye. Good vision in the one eye is not affected by cataract in the other. In order to make a decision about the need for surgery, a person should consider how much the cataract is interfering with her/his day-to-day activities. Obviously, a person who needs excellent eyesight for work will more than likely need surgery earlier than a person who doesn't.

What does cataract surgery involve?
In a sentence, the cloudy lens is removed by ultrasonic power and microsurgical techniques and then replaced by a new plastic implant. However, before the operation is performed, a patient's level of vision is tested, the eye is examined and measured to decide the strength of the lens needed. The operation itself is generally done under local anaesthetic.

Preparation for cataract surgery?
Cataract surgery is usually done as a day case, which means a patient is admitted and discharged on the same day, although only with an escort. Once a patient has been admitted to hospital, a nurse will put dilating drops into the eye and prepare the patient for operating theatre. A plastic needle, called 'a canula,' is normally inserted into the back of the hand by an anaesthetist, before the local anaesthetic is given to numb the eye. A patient lies flat during the operation with a single pillow under the head. The patient's face is covered with a sterile drape to keep the area clean. A patient must lie still for about thirty minutes, while the cataract is being removed. After the operation, the eye is covered with a shield and the patient is returned to the day ward.

What happens during cataract surgery?

- The eye is not removed from its socket during any kind of eye surgery. A small cut is made at the top or side of the eye, near the iris.

- An instrument, called a probe, is passed through the cut. A hole is made in the lens capsule covering the front surface of the cataract and the probe is passed into it. The probe breaks the cataract into very small pieces, which are sucked out of the eye. The remainder of the lens capsule, the clear outer covering of the cataract, is left in place.

- A plastic lens is used to replace the cataract. It's folded in half and inserted inside the lens capsule through the cut at the front of the eye. Once inside the lens capsule, the plastic lens unfolds to its normal shape.

- The small cut usually heals naturally

- After the operation, a pad or shield is placed over the eye.

What happens after cataract surgery?
After cataract surgery, a person can lead a normal life. S/he is given an appointment for a post-operative review and prescribed a course of eye drops. For about four weeks after the surgery, the patient must avoid lifting heavy objects, vacuuming, gardening, swimming, etc. In fact, a full list of DO's and DON'T's is given to each patient after cataract surgery. A patient will need to clean the eyelids each morning and drops must be put into the eye between four and six times a day, as prescribed, for about a month after the surgery. The drops prevent infection and reduce inflammation after surgery. The patient is advised to avoid rubbing and touching the eye and to wear a protective plastic shield in bed for about two weeks after the operation.

At the conclusion of a very informative, if unnerving, consultation, Mr Wallace prescribed a six-week course of saline drops and recommended that I return to Dr O'Regan for further review. On the way home, I stated to my wife, Sheila, who was to walk steadfastly by my side for the entirety of the medical journey ahead, that it looked like I was facing four eye surgeries in the years ahead.

"Yes" she replied. "You will need to have two cataract surgeries and two corneal transplants." When she added that the surgeries would be well spaced out and that I'd be in very good hands, I didn't feel one bit reassured.

CHAPTER FIVE

MONITORING MY VISION

On my return to Dr O'Regan for review a few weeks later, he provided me with a prescription for reading glasses as the cataracts were not at a stage where surgery was necessary nor advisable. His recommendation was to monitor the deterioration in my eyesight and then to consider cataract surgery at the most appropriate and beneficial time. It was very good advice and it provided me with a more tangible timeline and a greater self-belief in my ability to cope with what was to come. My understanding was that cataract surgery was available locally but that I would more than likely have to attend the Royal Victoria Eye and Ear Hospital in Dublin for the corneal transplant surgery. I found it useful to have all of that information at hand as it gave me some clarity about the medical procedures ahead of me. I also learned that Moorfield Eye Hospital, London which is Europe's largest centre for eye treatment and research, had an outstanding reputation in the type of surgery that I would soon require. When the time was right, I was ready and willing to attend Dublin or London on the recommendation of the medical specialists. As it turned out, it wasn't necessary for me to attend either Dublin or London as I became a beneficiary of good timing about eighteen months later. I'll go into that stoke of good luck in detail in Chapter Nine.

As 2018 progressed, I was coping very well with my new reading glasses, which was a great relief as I am an avid reader. I also have a great love of writing and am a regular contributor to a number of newspapers and magazines. My main area of commentary is in education, careers and the world of work as most of my professional life was spent in career and educational counselling. I am also a devoted sea swimmer and I acted as Secretary and PRO of our local swimming club, Tralee Swimming Club, for a long period of time until the club was formally dissolved at the Grand Hotel, Denny Street, Tralee on 4th October 2001 due to an alleged accident at the bathing slip in Fenit. The swimming club was wound-up almost fifty years after it had been founded at the same venue on 21st June 1952. In 2017, I published a book entitled, 'From Fenit bathing slip to the High Court - A five-year journey of honour!', which was launched by Martin Ferris TD at the Grand Hotel, Tralee, Co. Kerry on Monday, 8th May 2017. Deputy Ferris, who is a native of the Fenit area, played a significant role in saving the bathing slip in Fenit from demolition by the Department of Communications Marine and Natural Resources in 2004. In fact, the bathing slip would have been irrevocably lost to the swimming community of Kerry and the thousands of visitors who holiday in the region annually without the proactive support of Kerry's national and local public representatives. Written in first person narrative form, the book covered the glorious story of Tralee Swimming Club and its pivotal position in the sporting and social life of the community. I dealt with the reasons for the untimely dissolution of the club on 4th October 2001.

I explained in the book why the Government was determined to demolish the bathing slip in Fenit and how a public campaign was organised to save a priceless leisure facility in the picturesque village. The campaign was waged in a tenacious and persistent manner against the might of the State from 2001 to 2004 and took me into the corridors of power in Dublin. The three-year campaign captured the imagination and the overwhelming support of the general public and was wholeheartedly backed by the county's politicians, sports clubs and community groups. The campaign to save the bathing slip in Fenit was finally brought to a successful conclusion in the meeting chamber of Kerry County Council on the 18th October, 2004.

I went on to provide the reader with a fascinating insight into the legal case which took five years to run its course and went all the way to the High Court in Limerick on the 16th October 2006. From beginning to end the book provided the reader with a captivating narrative of a small rural swimming community's battle for its bathing slip and its good name.

Tralee Swimming Club was based in Fenit village situated about 12km north-west of Tralee. Fenit is a picturesque seaside village with excellent facilities for lovers of water sports, including swimming, sailing, rowing and fishing as well as for the thousands of people of all ages who enjoy a relaxing sojourn by the sea. For me, the jewel in the crown of the facilities at Fenit is the public bathing slip, which is located at the end of the path along the beach from the entrance to what is locally known as Locke's Beach. The history of the bathing slip and that of Tralee Swimming Club are inextricably intertwined. For almost fifty years, from 1952 to 2001, the swimming club was based at the bathing slip, which it maintained and upgraded on a voluntary basis. Prior to the advent of indoor swimming facilities, swimmers flocked to the bathing slip to enjoy a pleasant swim or to experience the thrill of jumping into the sea from the high and low diving boards. It is ironic that these same diving boards were indirectly and inculpably the cause of the dissolution of a wonderful club which provided such a healthy and enjoyable outlet for generations of swimmers.

As the last Secretary of Tralee Swimming Club, I felt under an obligation to write the history of Tralee Swimming Club and to record and chronicle the events which let all the way to the High Court in 2006. I was proud to have done so, despite my inability to do justice to the indefatigable efforts of the officers and members of the club, who contributed a life time of service to a facility which they dearly loved. Regardless of my own limitations as a writer, I felt it incumbent on me to record the story to perpetuate the memory of altruistic people and to acknowledge their contribution. I endeavoured in my research to uncover as much information about Tralee Swimming Club and to identify as many of the people as possible who have contributed to the story of Tralee Swimming Club, to the maintenance of the bathing slip, to the campaign to save the bathing slip at Fenit and finally to the High Court case in 2006. I felt it more comfortable to write the story in first person as I was a part of the story rather than a disinterested author who was looking in from outside. I felt it was important to record the events covered in the subject matter of the book in order to have a record of the period and to ensure that the glorious past of Tralee Swimming Club was never forgotten.

The book sold very well locally and I divided the net profit of €2,000 earned by the book equally between Spa/Fenit Youth Club at Fenit Parish Centre, Fenit, Tralee, in which area I live and Austin Stacks Juvenile GAA Club in my native Rock, Tralee, where I had very happy days and acquired values that stood me in good stead throughout my life.

Researching and writing the book gave me great pleasure and satisfaction. I learned a great deal about the difficulties encountered in publishing a book, why it's so difficult to find a publisher and why so many aspiring authors, like myself, are forced to take the lonely road of self-publishing a book. However, after my initial outing as an author, I was gripped by the writing bug and was determined to write a best-selling-novel.

In the summer of 2018, I scribbled down a few subject matters which were running through my head. I was confident that I had the ingredients for a good novel, which I was determined to have written and published in a calendar year. I wasn't certain that I had a year at my disposal before my need for eye surgery intervened, but I felt that working against the clock would keep me well and truly focussed on getting the novel on the bookshelves.

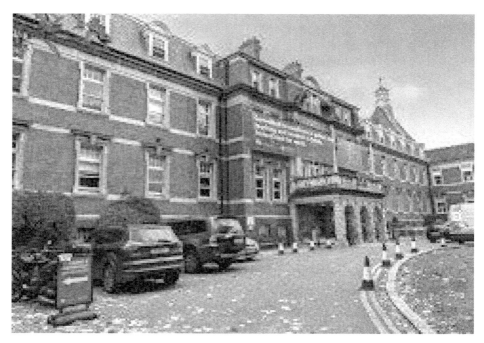
Royal Victoria Eye & Ear Hospital, Adelaide Road, Dublin 2

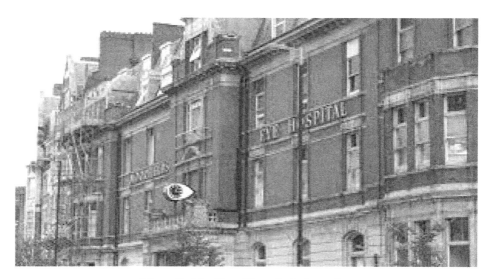
Moorfields Eye Hospital, London

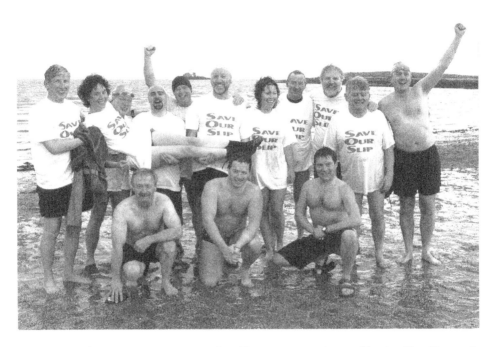

Save our Slip campaigners at the Christmas swim in Fenit, Co. Kerry in 2003 Back L/r Chris Nugent, Mags O Sullivan, Denis Cronin, John O Sullivan, Eddie Stack, Billy Ryle, Barbara O Sullivan, James O Herlihy, Paddy Kissane, John Paul Collins and Donal Fitzgibbon. Front L/r Liam Stack, Jack O Connor and Michael Martin

Photo courtesy of John Cleary

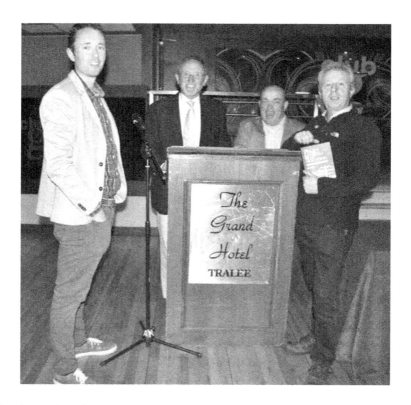

At the launch of Billy Ryle's history of Tralee Swimming Club at the Grand Hotel, Tralee on 8th May 2017 were L/r: Kevin Ryle, Billy Ryle, Kerry O'Shea and Éamonn O'Reilly

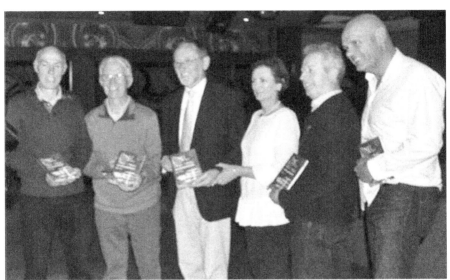

At the launch of Billy Ryle's history of Tralee Swimming Club at the Grand Hotel, Tralee on 8th May 2017 were Tommy O'Connor, Kerry County Librarian, Pat O'Mahony, Billy Ryle, Sheila Ryle, Éamonn O'Reilly and John Joe Sheehy

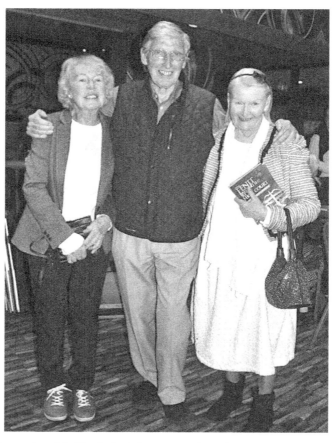

At the launch of Billy Ryle's history of Tralee Swimming Club at the Grand Hotel, Tralee on 8th May 2017 were L/r: Betty & Chris Nugent and Violet Ryle

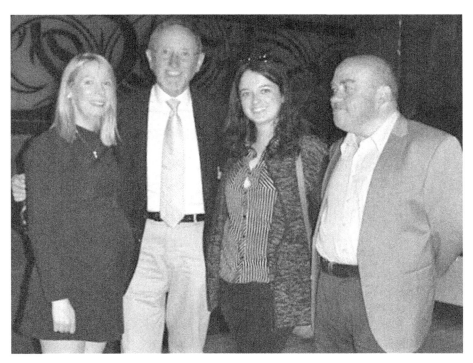

At the launch of Billy Ryle's history of Tralee Swimming Club at the Grand Hotel, Tralee on 8th May 2017 were L/r: Anne-Marie Ryle, Billy Ryle, Gráinne Ryle and Kerry O'Shea

CHAPTER SIX

CAMPAIGN FOR DIVING BOARDS

In 2017, I became very involved in a campaign to restore the diving boards at the bathing slip in Fenit. Back in 2004, when Kerry County Council took responsibility for the upkeep of the bathing slip, the restoration of the diving boards was excluded from the agreement. That was a compromise which had to made at the time in order to secure the future of the bathing slip. However, it was always my intention to raise the issue of restoring the diving boards when the time was right. The opportunity arose at the local launch of my book, 'From Fenit bathing slip to the High Court – a five-year journey of honour,' at Fenit Parish Hall on Friday, 19th May 2017. I stated that the diving boards had to be restored as a matter of urgency at the public bathing slip in Fenit. I informed the large attendance at the event, which was hosted by Fenit and Spa Youth Club, that the diving boards had a magnetic appeal, particularly for young swimmers. During the previous fifteen years, footfall at the bathing slip had decreased considerably due to the loss of the high and low diving boards. A generation of young people had missed out on the thrill of diving at the bathing slip. I told my audience that a magnificent marina had been established on the Pier in Fenit a few years earlier by laying a foundation of rock armour on the sea bed and building the infrastructure on it.

"Using similar engineering and construction principles," I said, "the bathing slip can be extended about 40m into deep water, thereby guaranteeing permanent and adequate water depth for swimming and spring board diving." I added that Fenit was now a major tourist destination and ever-increasing numbers were enjoying a summer holiday in the area.

As a result of my appeal, a committee from Fenit Development Association was established for the expressed purpose of having the diving boards restored at the bathing slip. After eighteen months of widespread consultation and research, a planning application for diving boards at Fenit bathing slip was lodged with Kerry County Council on behalf of Fenit Development Association on 30th November 2018.

Since the project had been given the full backing of Kerry County Council at a meeting between the sides on the 18th April 2018, the committee had been busy finalising the design with due regard to local tidal and weather conditions. The project was also designed to meet the standards and safety requirements of Kerry County Council and Irish Water Safety. The project was completely community based, so the entire cost of the work would, hopefully, be met by grant aid and a local contribution. The new diving boards would be an entirely public free-to-use aqua-sports facility and would include disability access.

We were delighted that the planning application for the diving boards had now been lodged with the planning authority. We were confident that the application would travel trouble free through the planning process and we were hoping to have good news for the huge crowd that would gather on Christmas morning for Fenit's annual Christmas Day swim.

We were very grateful to Kerry County Council which had pledged every possible advisory support during the construction of the diving boards. When the project was completed, Kerry County Council, which owns the property, would include the diving boards in its foreshore licence and insurance cover and would maintaining the bathing slip to the highest standard. We were extremely grateful to Malachy Walsh and Partners, Engineering & Environmental Consultants for their professionalism and expertise in designing diving boards which would stand the test of time at the bathing slip. We were indebted to the local sporting organisations and the general public for their support and goodwill for the project. The five people who led the campaign since July 2017 and who successfully negotiated with Kerry County Council – Mike O'Neill, Liam Doyle, Paddy Kissane, John Edwards and myself – would continue to oversee the project right through to completion. It was the committee's intention to begin construction work on the site as soon as possible after planning permission had been granted. Now that the planning application had been lodged with Kerry County Council, we were confident that Fenit was one step closer to the restoration of a much loved and badly missed sports and leisure facility which would have considerable sporting, social, economic, tourism and recreational value.

Unfortunately, two separate objections were lodged with Kerry County Council. The first objection was received by Kerry County Council on 3rd January 2019. The second objection was lodged with Kerry County Council on 10th January 2019. Each and every issue raised in the objections was addressed in a comprehensive and detailed response to Kerry County Council by Malachy Walsh and Partners, Engineering & Environmental Consultants, Blennerville, Tralee, Co. Kerry on behalf of Fenit Development Association.

On 20th August 2019, Fenit Development Association was informed by Kerry County Council that a grant of permission authorising the development would be granted after four weeks from that date provided no objection was lodged with An Bord Pleanala. Fenit Development Association welcomed the decision by Kerry County Council of 20th August 2019 to grant planning permission for the development of diving boards at the Bathing Slip, Fenit, Co. Kerry. As expected by Fenit Development Association, a further objection was lodged with An Bord Pleanala against the granting of planning permission.

We were resolute in our conviction that the decision of Kerry County Council to grant planning permission for the development of the diving boards was arrived at after a robust, professional and detailed inspection of Fenit Development Association's planning application. Fenit Development Association was confident that An Bord Pleanala would uphold the decision of Kerry County Council. Fenit Development Association cooperated fully with An Bord Pleanala and was very pleased to furnish it with whatever written, visual or oral submissions it requested.

Fenit Development Association again expressed its gratitude to Kerry County Council, owners of the Bathing Slip in Fenit, for consenting to include the diving boards in its foreshore licence and insurance cover and for agreeing to maintain the bathing slip to the highest standard. The project was designed for and would be developed for the benefit of the greater good of the general public, both locals and visitors. The project would create a Blue Space, which would provide access for all abilities to participate in aqua sports. The new diving boards and bathing slip area would be an entirely public free-to-use aqua-sports facility and would include disability access. The diving boards project would be an integral component of the overall plan for the development of tourism and leisure infrastructure in Fenit. It would provide the region with one of the finest facilities of its type in Europe and it would have considerable social, economic, tourism and recreational added value on the North Kerry Blue Way. It would provide a centre of swimming and diving excellence at the Bathing Slip in Fenit. It would be another major step on the road to having Tralee Bay designated as a National Centre for Aquatic Sports. Fenit Development Association thanked the general public for its wholehearted support and good wishes for this unique project. We expressed our indebtedness to the many swimmers and bathers in Fenit, both regulars and visitors, who expressed support for the project.

Fenit Development was confident that An Bord Pleanala would uphold the decision of Kerry County Council to grant planning permission for the restoration of the diving boards. The quality of the information which we had submitted to Kerry County Council and subsequently to An Bord Pleanala, was of an exceptional standard. Nevertheless, there is always an element of doubt about the outcome of these matters. An Bord Pleanala carried out a forensic examination of our submission and that of the objectors. It was well over a year before they issued their decision in our favour on 18th December 2020, subject to the following five conditions.

1. The development shall be carried out and completed in accordance with the plans and particulars lodged with the application, as amended by the further plans and particulars submitted on the 29th day of January 2019 and the 24th July 2019, and by the further plans and particulars received by An Bord Pleanála on the 15th October 2019 and the 6th April 2020, except as may otherwise be required in order to comply with the following conditions. Where such conditions require details to be agreed with the planning authority, the developer shall agree such details in writing with the planning authority prior to commencement of development and the development shall be carried out and completed in accordance with the agreed particulars.
   Reason: In the interest of clarity.

2. The proposed development shall be amended as follows: (a) The ramp and the lower pillar/platform/diving board shall be omitted. (b) An additional ladder shall be installed on the eastern side of the retained higher pillar/platform. (c) The wall and fence proposed for the western side of the walkway shall be omitted in favour of railings. Revised drawings showing compliance with these requirements shall be submitted to, and agreed in writing with, the planning authority prior to commencement of development.
   Reason: In the interests of amenity and public safety.

3. The Mitigation Measures as set out in Chapter 10 of the Natura Impact Statement, which was submitted to An Bord Pleanala on the 6th day of April 2020, shall be implemented in full.
   Reason: In the interest of the protection of the environment.

4. The construction of the development shall be managed in accordance with a Construction Management Plan, which shall be submitted to, and agreed in writing with, the planning authority prior to commencement of development. This plan shall provide

details of intended construction practice and access arrangements for the development. The Plan shall also state the projected construction period and the tidal ranges that would occur during the days comprised in this period. ABP-305431-19 Board Direction Page 4 of 4

Reason: In the interests of clarity, public safety, and orderly and well-planned development.

5. Prior to the commencement of use of the diving facility, the railings to the walkway and the ladders to the platform shall be installed and the colour code system to the pillar shall be in place. Thereafter, these items shall be retained in-situ for the duration of the use of this diving facility.

   Reason: In the interest of public safety.

Mike O' Neill, Chairman of Fenit Development Association welcomed the decision by An Bord Pleanala to grant permission for the restoration of diving boards at Fenit after an absence of twenty-five years. Mike stated that the decision meant that Fenit would have a fully functional and safe outdoor-diving facility available to the public during the summer months when the tides are favourable.

"The boards will add hugely to Fenit as a fun, healthy and sustainable activity for visitors and locals alike," Mike added. "It will be a great boost for the swimming community and will add to the Blue Space in Fenit and when added to The Greenway and all of the other outdoor pursuits available in the area it will help make Fenit a premier destination for all lovers of the great outdoors. This positive decision represents over three years of work by the committee and the project will be finished to the highest building and safety standards guaranteeing fun diving for the next fifty years. We would like to thank Kerry County Council for granting planning permission and also for their support in the early stages of the project. We would also like to thank the people of Fenit who have supported the proposal from the outset and also a big thanks to all swimmers who have shown support over the years. The positive decision represents a real antidote to a really tough year for so many people and we can finally say that our boards are coming back."

I was overjoyed by the decision of An Bord Pleanála. It had taken three years of dedicated and sustained work by the five of us to have reached this critical stage. The objections had considerably delayed our progress and had cost a great deal of extra expenditure in responding to the objections. This was money which could more productively have been spent on the construction of the diving boards. But it was well worth it and the process validated the quality of our planning application. Fenit Development Association also accepted the legal entitlement of any individual or organisation to object to a planning application. In our case, we bore no ill feeling towards the individuals whose names were on the documents of objection. When the diving boards are in position, all of the objectors without exception will be more than welcome to enjoy this unique facility at the bathing slip.

In December 2020, when the good news about the diving boards was made public, my eye sight was irreversibly deteriorating. Just a year before in December 2019, I had had cataract surgery in my right eye and it was only a matter of time before a similar procedure would follow in my left eye. The inevitability of two corneal transplants of donor organs filled me with apprehension.

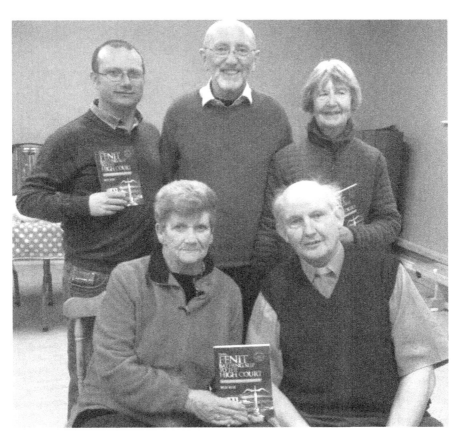

At the local launch of Billy Ryle's history of Tralee Swimming Club at the Parish Centre in Fenit, Co. Kerry on the 19th May 2017 were Front L/r Kathleen Murphy and Fr Denis O'Mahony Back L/r: Aidan Murphy, Billy Ryle and Margaret Crowley

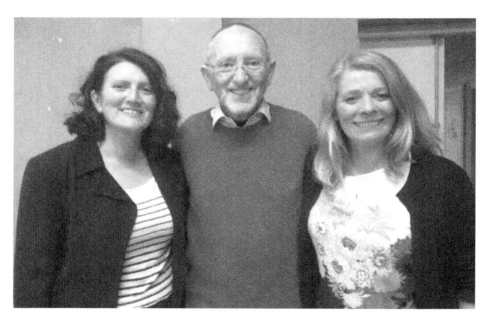

At the local launch of Billy Ryle's history of Tralee Swimming Club at the Parish Centre in Fenit, Co. Kerry on the 19th May 2017 were L/r: Mary Tobin, Billy Ryle and Máire Vieux

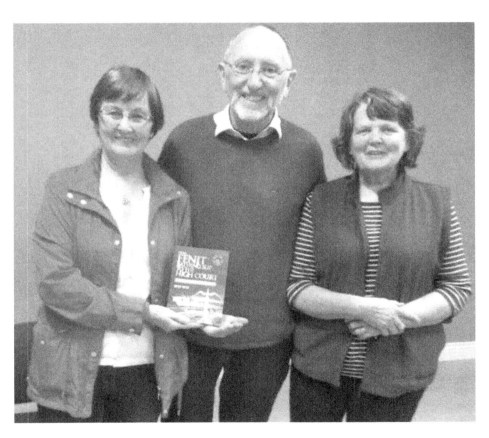

At the local launch of Billy Ryle's history of Tralee Swimming Club at the Parish Centre in Fenit, Co. Kerry on the 19th May 2017 were L/r: Mary Jo Walsh, Billy Ryle and Catherine Moriarty

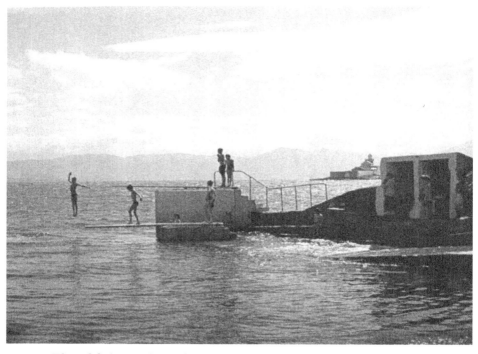
The old diving boards at the Bathing Slip, Fenit, Co. Kerry

CHAPTER SEVEN

THE BENEFITS OF SEA SWIMMING

As I mentioned earlier, I began researching material for a novel during the summer of 2018. By this stage I wasn't wearing glasses other than for reading. This was a new situation for me as I had been wearing bifocal glasses for many years. But with cataract and cornea problems developing in both eyes, distance lens were no longer of any benefit to me. I was still attending most of the Austin Stack football matches, but I was beginning to position myself on the terrace directly opposite the halfway line. That vantage point allowed me to follow the game with some degree of visual comfort although I was beginning to have some difficulty in identifying players on the far corners of the field.

Other than the diagnosis of the health problems with my eyes, 2018 was a very fulfilling year for me. Swimming conditions in Fenit were ideal and the weather during the year was conducive to outdoor living. I prefer an early morning swim as it gets the day off to a good start. If there is sufficient water in the bathing slip, I usually swim around 9am with the regular swimmers who follow the tide. The walk along the path from the carpark in Fenit to the bathing slip offers a scenic route of aerobic exercise to me and my faithful canine companion, Jake, who is a golden cocker spaniel with a lovely temperament and a passion for exercise. As a personal who prefers to swim in the sea rather than to take a long walk, my routine allows me to kill two birds with one stone. Jake rejoices in his exercise to and from the bathing slip, which I also enjoy. But it's a different matter when I jump into the deep clear water of Tralee Bay. I am a natural swimmer who feels very much at home in sea water. I have a great respect for the sea and the good practices for safe swimming in the ocean. I always swim parallel to the shore and remain close enough to shore to make it safely to dry land in the event of a cramp or some unforeseen illness or mishap. I always swim with my companions for safety in numbers and for the fun and craic that comes from good company in our chat and banter before and after the swim. As deep water at the bathing slip is tidal dependent where full tide is about an hour later each day, it's not always possible to swim every morning. While I prefer the morning swim, an afternoon swim causes only minor inconvenience to me as I always set aside an hour or so in my schedule to go for my dip and to take Jake for his daily exercise.

There is something very special about swimming in seawater. The physical and mental health benefits of open water swimming are considerable, When I was younger, I loved the competitive swims which kept me super fit and sharpened my edge for success. I really enjoyed the middle-distance swims where I had the time to enjoy the sea in all its moods and transitions. I developed a strategy to take advantage of the favourable currents, to conserve energy when swimming against the tide, to avoid the serpentine rip tides and, of course, to have enough juice in the tank for the speedy swim to the line. It was always good for the ego and the self-confidence to finish in a medal position.

In recent years, I have become a dedicated aerobic non-competitive swimmer and do my best to enjoy a daily swim, weather permitting. The anticipation of the swim, in itself, gives me a very positive fillip. It helps me to better organise and to get the most out of every day. The endorphin rush that comes from engaging with the sea is a wonderful experience.

A good swim is one of the easiest ways to release endorphins. The more you swim, the more endorphins your body will produce. Athletes often talk about feeling a 'runner's high' after a good run. I experience the same high after a good dip in the sea, where my efforts result in an explosive release of endorphins. All my aches and pains just seem to dissolve when I'm swimming. My daily swim keeps me in good form and in a positive frame of mind. If I ever get into the sea with any of the stress and anxiety that comes with daily living, I'm totally relaxed and at peace with the world when I emerge from the water. I'm overcome by feelings of wellbeing and contentment. Swimming has also given me a high level of self-confidence and a balanced attitude to life. I consider myself to be a good-humoured and compassionate person with an ability to cope with the ups and downs of life. Swimming has been a great outlet for me in my battle with Fuchs Dystrophy during the last few years.

I have been an all-year-round swimmer for many years. There is something cathartic and energising about the feel of cold sea water. A winter swim is an invigorating experience. There is a spiritual dimension to it. It brings me closer to the many wonders of nature and the Divine Being who provided such a wonderful world for mankind. During the two-year Covid-19 lockdown and isolation, the sea was my faithful friend as it was to the swimming community. It brought purpose to each day and while my normal social interaction was restricted, I always had the outlet of swimming in the deep blue ocean. The winter swim is much shorter and a lot less time is spent in the water, but that doesn't matter at all. The benefits are every bit as precious as a summer swim in the warm water on the Costa del Sol on a hot July day. Having said that, I must admit that I really look forward to a week of warm water swimming in Spain each April and again in September every year!

I am a strong advocate of aerobic exercise for people of all ages but particularly for older people. My sport of choice is swimming, but a daily walk or jog, a game of racquet sport or whatever form of exercise a person enjoys is very worthwhile, both physically and mentally. Its only when something happens to disrupt your routine that you appreciate what you have and what you are at risk of losing. I had been living the good life without a care in the world when my eye disease was diagnosed. The inner strength that I had acquired from swimming and my Catholic faith gave me the resolve and determination to face the journey ahead.

CHAPTER EIGHT

THE NOVEL

It's often said that there is a novel in every person and successful writers advise newcomers to write about what they know. I took that advice to heart when I decided to tackle my unfulfilled ambition of writing a novel. A novel by definition is a work of fiction and it allows the writer to be very creative and imaginative. This genre was a new experience for me. As my writing experience so far was based around education and sport, the style was factual, reportage, narrative and informational. I had also taken an online course in Journalism with the Irish Academy of Public Relations, which was very interesting and informative and provided me with a very useful insight into writing styles. I was already very influenced by one of my favourite authors, Jeffrey Archer, who maintains that a good novel is a gripping story which keeps the reader turning the pages.

So, during summer 2018, I made a tentative start on a novel which was a work of fiction but dealt with many of the issues that I encountered during my teenage years. The hero in the book is Barry Kyle, talented footballer, keen student, altar server, republican and loyal friend, who lives in the fictious town of Tradinveen, Co. Kerry. His parents, Jack and Jill Kyle run a pub and grocery shop. Jack is a community leader, a problem solver, Chairman of Rockfield GAA Club, Roman Catholic and IRA Official. Jack and Jill have four children – Mary, Barry, Mark and Paul, an orphan adopted from the 'The Industrial.' Barry's best friend John is a homosexual.

Barry attends the local Mercy Primary School from 1954 to 1958. His friendship with Brother Ambrose, gifted teacher and skilful Gaelic football coach, develops at 'The Small Mon' from 1958 to 1963. Barry transfers to 'The Big Mon' in 1963 where he encounters the traditional Brother Thomas, who is determined to win The Moran Cup. Barry suffers ongoing bullying from Bobby Collins, Vice-Principal, Free Stater and bitter enemy of the republican Kyle family since the Irish Civil War.

The Christian Brothers have high academic expectations of Barry. They are keen for Barry to become a Christian Brother. The Dominican's expect Barry to follow in the footsteps of his great-uncle Fr. Don Kyle OP while Fr. O Brien PP wants Barry to transfer to the Diocesan Seminary, 'The Dice' in Killarney. The Big Mon and The Dice are bitter rivals. Meanwhile, Brother Ambrose, who has set up a very progressive juvenile football structure in Rockfield GAA Club, is a positive constant in Barry's adolescent life and stands up to be counted when John's homosexuality is exposed.

Many of the contemporary issues of the period – brutality, corporal punishment, Catholicism, The Irish Language, republicanism, homosexuality, adoption, The Industrial School, bullying, murder, assassination, GAA, IRA, post-Civil War tension, etc are seamlessly embroidered into this compelling story.

The story follows Barry's adolescent conflict between his religious vocation and his developing sexuality. It draws in many of the seminal events and personalities of the period – John Fitzgerald Kennedy, Martin Luther King, Jack Lynch, Donogh O Malley, the permissive '60's, Hippies, Flower Power generation, etc. The book captures the ambiguity, bigotry and hypocrisy of a time, when Barry's brother, Paul is called 'a bastard from The Industrial' and his best friend John is called 'a fucking pervert.'

I had the first draft of the novel written by Christmas 2018 and in the new year I set about finding a company to publish my book. I received a few tentative expressions of interest but I soon began to realise that book publishing companies were reluctant to take on an unknown author. I began to look at other publishing options. I took some consolation from a statement once made by the wonderful Maeve Binchy to the effect that she got ten rejections before securing a publisher for her first novel, Light a Penny Candle, which went on to become an international bestseller! My remaining options were to self-publish or to engage with Amazon. Eventually, I decided to go the Amazon route which was not as clear cut as I had expected. I was under the illusion that Amazon would provide proof reading, editing, design, publication in print and digital as well as distribution of the printed book. Amazon did publish the book and print the number of copies which I ordered and was asked to pay for in advance. Although the people I dealt with were very helpful and encouraging, Amazon didn't provide an editing facility nor a distribution service. My order of paperback copies of the book was delivered to my home address. While Amazon provides an author with a potential worldwide readership of the digital book and an online book purchase platform, it's not as good for a new author as having the support of a publishing and distributing company.

The Book could, and still can, be purchased online from Amazon. A digital e-book version (kindle) is also available from Amazon. Thanks to the generosity of local bookshops and shops in my home area of Spa and Fenit, my book was available for purchase at €12 per copy. I was very grateful to the business premises which facilitated the sale of my book as the revenue earned was a great help in covering the cost of producing the book. In addition, there was a huge turnout at the official launch of the book by Declan Malone, former Editor of The Kerryman Newspaper at Kerry Library, Moyderwell, Tralee on Thursday, 13th June 2019. Popular Tralee man, Kerry O'Shea, Reporter with Outlook Magazines was Master of Ceremonies at the Book launch. I was overjoyed by the success of the launch and pleasantly surprised by the number of people who purchased copies of the book.

I began my brief address at the launch by welcoming everybody and thank them for attending. I thanked Kerry County Librarian, Tommy O Connor for hosting the launch at Tralee Library on that particular night. My thanks also went to Tommy, Patti Ann O Leary and John O Connell for their invaluable assistance in organising and preparing the venue.

"I'm delighted that the launch is taking place in the Library, where I regularly spend time browsing through the book shelves. The Library is always a hub of activity and I'd like to compliment Tommy and his colleagues in the Library Branches throughout the county for their outstanding work in encouraging people of all ages to read.

I'm thrilled to have written my first novel. I once learned in a workshop that its best to write about what you know. I took my inspiration for this novel from my wonderful youthful years of football with the Austin Stacks GAA Club, Tralee and ten years of outstanding education from the Christian Brothers. I enjoyed the freedom to be imaginative and creative while writing this work of fiction.

This novel took me into the jungles of Africa, to the back streets of Lima, to the hippy colony of San Francisco, to St. Peters Square in Rome, to the missions of Trinidad, to Hill 16 in Croke Park, to the Quays of Waterford, where Edmund Ignatius Rice founded the Christian Brothers, whose record in fostering Catholicism, Republicanism, Gaelic Games and the Irish language is unequalled. It allowed me to comment on the political and social histories of the swinging 1960's and embroider some of the major issues of the day into the story. My football teams, coached by Brother Ambrose and Brother Thomas played fast attacking football. Was that style of football good enough to restore the glory days to the CBS Secondary School, popularly known as The Big Mon?

Kerry O Shea knows the answer to that question because he has spent the past week reading the novel. Kerry is a great friend. Every time I speak with Kerry, I learn something new. When it comes to Kerry and Rock football there is very little that he doesn't know. He travels the length and breadth of the country reporting on his beloved Kerry. Like myself, he has great affection for the Austin Stacks GAA Club. He was a vital member of the editorial team which spent two years researching and writing the Austin Stacks Centenary Book and his forensic coverage of The First Golden Era of the Rock Club from 1928 to 1936 is iconic. His Tralee Town News in Outlook Magazines has a huge readership and Kerry is a popular man about town. I appreciate having Kerry as Master of Ceremonies this evening

I'm very grateful to Declan Malone for coming in from Dingle to launch my novel. Declan is a very distinguished journalist, who worked in The Kerryman for twenty-seven years, fifteen of them as Editor. His instinct for a good story and his keen sense of community makes him an outstanding journalist. His writing is incisive, interesting, informative, balanced and objective without ever being intrusive or offensive.

Declan guided The Kerryman safely through the many challenges presented by the advent of social media. He oversaw the transfer of headquarters from Clash Industrial Estate to Denny Street in 2007 and he facilitated the change from broadsheet to compact format in 2008.

 In 2015, he surprised everybody when he announced that he was retiring as Editor to spend more time fishing off Ventry Harbour. However, Declan hasn't been completely lost to journalism as his weekly West Kerry column has added a very colourful dimension to The Kerryman. His coverage of community activities and his creative photo journalism lets no one in doubt that Dingle is the capital of adventure, culture, music and the good life.

Declan is closely associated with Hope Guatemala, a West Kerry based charity, which is active at grassroots level in Guatemala. It's comprised of volunteers only, with no management or administration costs. Its activities are funded solely through the efforts of volunteers with no Government funding involved. Its mission is to aid development and to support poverty relief in Guatemala. It has ten specific aims. The first of those is to feed fifty children twice a day and to pay for their medical care.

Declan declined my offer of a fee to launch my novel this evening. So, in anticipation of selling a few copies of my Book here this evening, I'd like to present Declan with €500 for the children of Guatemala. That money will do far more-good for the poor children of Guatemala than it will burning a hole in my pocket." Local media outlets were very generous with the coverage given to the launch and I also did some advertising to boost sales. In the end, I just about covered my expenses and often wondered would I have had a best seller on my hands if I'd had a publisher to promote and distribute the book to a much wider readership.

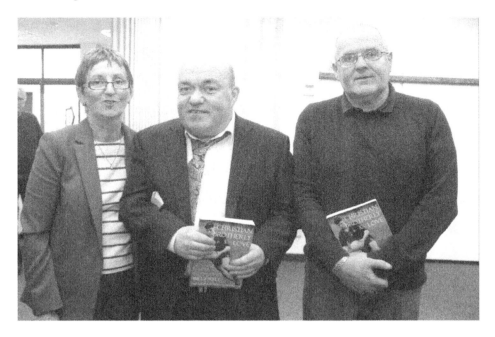

At the launch of Billy Ryle's novel, Christian Brotherly Love at Tralee Branch, Kerry County Library on the 13th June 2019 were L/r: Phil Dunne, Kerry O'Shea and Paudie Commane

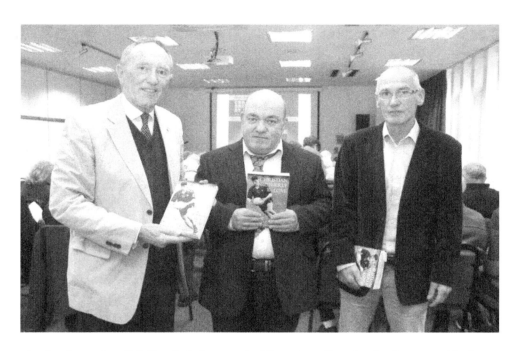

At the launch of Billy Ryle's novel, Christian Brotherly Love at Tralee Branch, Kerry County Library on the 13th June 2019 were L/r Billy Ryle, Kerry O'Shea and Declan Malone

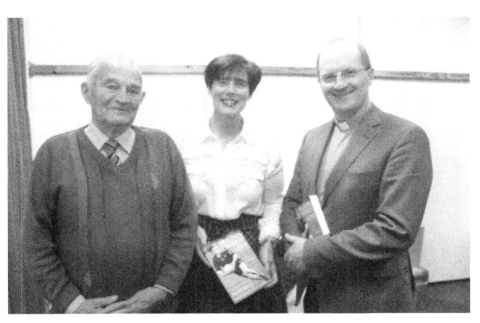

At the launch of Billy Ryle's novel, Christian Brotherly Love at Tralee Branch, Kerry County Library on the 13th June 2019 were L/r: Micheál Hayes, Norma Foley and Fr Pádraig Walsh

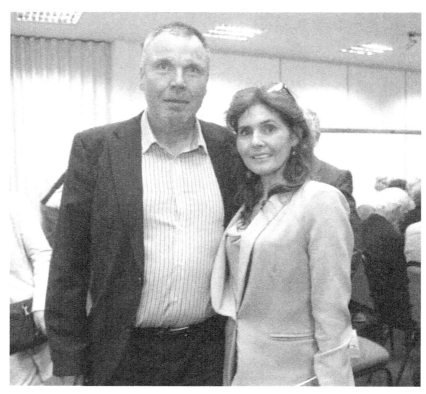

Nigel and Mary Crowe attended the launch of Billy Ryle's novel, Christian Brotherly Love at Tralee Branch, Kerry County Library on the 13th June 2019

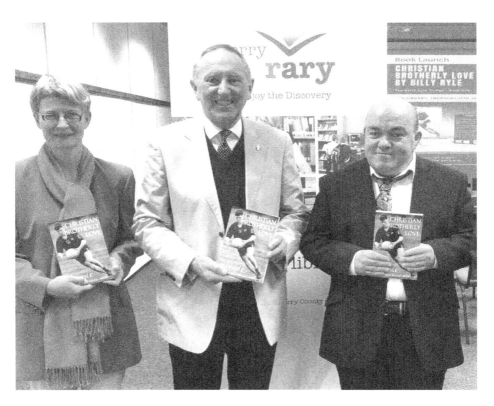

At the launch of Billy Ryle's novel, Christian Brotherly Love at Tralee Branch, Kerry County Library on the 13th June 2019 were L/r Patty Anne O'Leary, Librarian, Billy Ryle and Kerry O'Shea

CHAPTER NINE

NEW CONSULTANT OPHTHALMIC SURGEON

In the Autumn of 2019, Dr O'Regan contacted me to let me know that a new Consultant appointment had recently been made at Bon Secours Hospital Cork. Dr O'Regan furnished me with some biographical information about Mr Tom Flynn, Consultant Ophthalmic Surgeon, who had taken up the appointment. It made for very impressive reading. I went on to read that Mr Flynn graduated as a Doctor from University College Cork in 1999 and began his ophthalmology training in Cork. He moved to London in 2004 where he was awarded a Doctoral Degree (PhD) for research on corneal transplant immunology at Moorfields Eye Hospital/University College London, Europe's largest centre for eye treatment and research. He undertook higher specialist and senior fellowship training at Moorfields. He had been a Consultant Ophthalmic Surgeon at Moorfields since 2013, specialising in the anterior segment of the eye – cornea, cataract and laser eye surgery. The document said that Mr Flynn's commitment to providing high-quality patient care had been recognised through Clinical Excellence Awards. His cataract surgery outcomes, as reported by the UK National Ophthalmology Database, were consistently better than the UK consultant national average. He has trained surgeons from all over the world and has published widely. His researched has influenced local and national policies e.g., hurling related eye injuries were significantly reduced as a result of early research he carried out in Cork.

The document stated that cataract surgery and corneal transplantation for keratoconus, infection, scarring and Fuchs Dystrophy were included in the areas of special interest for Mr Flynn. This information immediately grabbed my interest. Not only was Mr Flynn one of the leading experts in his area of specialisation, but now my cataract and corneal transplant surgeries could be carried out in Cork. I was thrilled with this development as I had studied for my BA HDE and Diploma in Guidance & Counselling at UCC as well as working in Cork for one academic year. I have a great affinity with Cork and always enjoy going into the city for GAA games and a bit of therapeutic shopping. During my student days in UCC, I had been a patient at Bon Secours Hospital, Cork when I required treatment for a leg injury. My four children Kevin, Gráinne, Brian and the late Aisling were all born in the Maternity Unit at the Bons. Kevin, Gráinne and Brian had also studied for their undergraduate degrees in Medicine, Pharmacy and Dentistry, respectively, at UCC.

From a logistical perspective, Cork was far more convenient than Dublin. The journey from my home at Spa Village to Cork normally took about two hours. With the new Macroom by-pass scheduled to open in the next few years, the journey would become even shorter. At this stage, my wife Sheila was doing all our long-distance driving and I knew that I could depend on her to accompany me to Cork whenever she was free to do so. On the occasions when I didn't have a driver, I had an excellent train and bus service at my disposal in Tralee. As Mr Flynn had based his Eye Clinic at Affidea, The Elysian, Eglinton Street, Cork, I would have only about a ten-minute walk to the Clinic from Kent Railway Station in Glanmire, Cork on days when I travelled to Cork by train.

Being of an age where I have free travel on all public transport, I was able to journey by train to Cork without having to pay. I had never before had occasion to utilise my free travel pass but I soon realised what a wonderful concession it is for those who have to make regular journeys. On my train travels, I met many people who, like myself, were travelling to Cork and Dublin for medical treatment. I spoke with students who had a daily round-trip commute from home to college. I had chats with elderly people on their way to Cork and Dublin for a day's shopping or to touch base with their children and grandchildren. I must commend Irish Rail for the courtesy and kindness of its staff. I was very impressed by the assistance given to disabled and elderly people. The trains were always clean, comfortable and warm and were invariably running on time. My experience over the past few years has made me a fan of and even an advocate for public transport.

I had some idea in my head that The Elysian was or had been the tallest building in Cork so my natural curiosity forced me to look it up. The literature stated that The Elysian is a mixed-use Celtic Tiger-era building at Eglinton Street, Cork. Construction of the building was completed in early September 2008. Built as part of a vision to redefine city living in Cork, the Elysian is a landmark development in the renewal of the south docklands area. Six to eight-storey buildings make up the majority of the complex, housing a mix of apartments, retail and commercial space arranged around a central garden courtyard. When built the 18-storey tower, at 68 metres-high, was the tallest building in the Republic of Ireland. It was overtaken by Capital Dock in the Dublin Docklands in 2018. The Elysian is an iconic marker for the surrounding city and suburbs. I had often seen the building in the distance but when I saw it up close and personal for the first time, I was very impressed. Tom Flynn Eye Clinic is on the ground floor section, known as Affidea, alongside a very convenient indoor car park.

I assume that The Elysian name was adapted from Elysium, also called Elysian Fields or Elysian Plain, in Greek mythology, which was originally the paradise to which heroes on whom the gods conferred immortality were sent. In Homer's writings the Elysian Plain was a land of perfect happiness at the end of the Earth, on the banks of the Oceanus, the river that flowed around the Earth. Only those especially favoured by the gods entered Elysium and were made immortal. When I entered The Elysian for the first time, I wasn't looking for immortality. I was hoping that my patron Saint, Martin De Porres OP, the Black Friar of Lima, in whom I have great faith, would protect me and keep me strong during my ordeal. I'm not certain if Saint Martin played any part in Mister Flynn's decision to return to Cork. Saint Martin has always delivered for me when I requested a favour. I try not to torment him too often. But I was now asking St Martin to keep a protective eye on proceedings as Mister Flynn set about restoring my eyesight to a functional level.

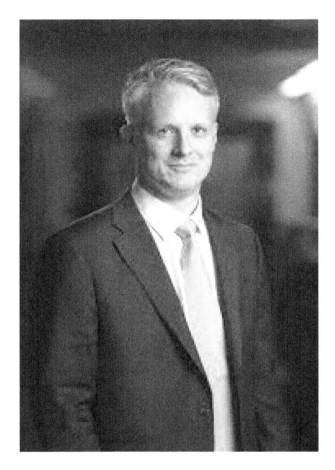

Mr Tom Flynn, Consultant Ophthalmic Surgeon

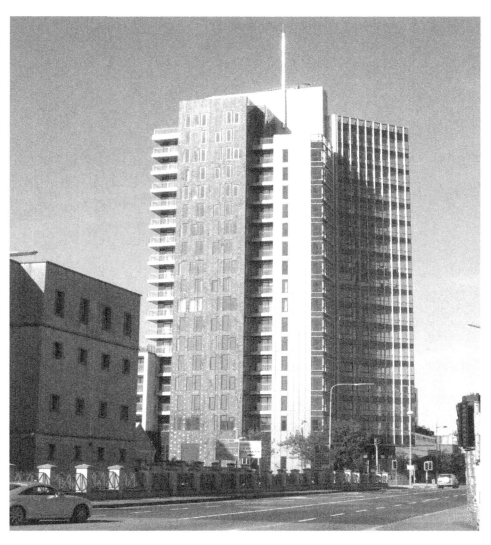

The Elysian Tower, Eglinton Street, Cork

CHAPTER TEN

RIGHT EYE CATARACT SURGERY

My first appointment with Mister Flynn was confirmed for 1.30pm on the 13th November, 2019 at the Outpatients Department, Bon Secours Hospital, College Road, Cork as Mister Flynn's Rooms, at The Elysian, weren't yet ready for consultations following his recent return to Cork from London. I travelled to Cork by train and as I had time on my hands before my appointment, I enjoyed a leisurely walk from Kent Station to the Bons. On my way, I stopped off to visit the UCC campus, where I had spent many happy years as a student. I dropped into the Honan Chapel on Connaught Avenue to say a prayer for a good outcome of my first meeting with Mister Flynn and any further medical procedures I might be facing.

During my time at UCC, there was a tradition that a final year student assisted the College Chaplin in preparing the altar and organising the altar servers for the Masses in the Honan Chapel. The title of *Bishop* went with this voluntary position which I was offered in my graduate year. The greatest difficulty I faced was in getting servers for first Mass at 8am. There was no such problem with the 1pm and 6pm Masses where the servers were keen to impress the large female attendance. A major perk of being Bishop was having first choice of altar serving the many visiting priests who said Mass in the Honan Chapel. The secular priests from the USA, Britain and Australia were very generous with their tips but the missionary priests from South America, The Philippines and Africa were as poor as the people to whom they devoted their lives. Other great memories from those youthful days were summers in England and the USA, where my education and mind were really broadened.

Student life in Cork was brilliant but I had one regrettable setback, which still haunts me. When I was a pupil at CBS Secondary School, The Green, Tralee my neighbour May Sugrue, who ran a little grocery shop, recruited me to deliver the morning milk in our area and to do some grocery deliveries on Saturday afternoon. I saved up to purchase a fabulous Raleigh bicycle from Jim Caball Himself, one of the town's popular bicycle shops. That bike carried me to school, to football, to basketball, to the library, to Fenit and to Banna, everywhere in fact. It transported me around Cork for nearly four years until, one day, I forgot to lock it before going into Woolworth's in Patrick St. The bicycle was gone when I came out. It took me a long time to get over the loss of my loyal companion and I never forgave myself for condemning my bicycle to permanent exile in Rebel country!

Anyway, when I arrived at the Bons in Cork, I asked for directions to the Outpatients Department. The Hospital had expanded considerably since I had last visited for the birth of my youngest son, Brian and it was a hive of activity. The outpatients' waiting room was full to capacity so I thought I was in for a long wait until it dawned on me that Mister Flynn was not the only Consultant seeing patients. After a short interval, my name was called and I was escorted into the Eye rooms. Mister Flynn and I had a discussion about my problem and he carried out a detailed examination of my eyes. Mister Flynn very kindly agreed to take me on as a patient and assured me that he would carry out the surgical procedures required to mitigate the problems with my eyesight. A follow up appointment was made for me to see Mr Flynn at his clinic at The Elysian on 6th December 2019.

Mr Flynn confirmed the diagnosis of bilateral cataracts and Fuchs Dystrophy. He told me that my gradual deterioration in vision and some diurnal fluctuation in vision was largely due to cataract but that I had obvious endothelial changes of Fuchs Dystrophy, which is a build up of fluid in the cornea on the front of the eye, causing the cornea to swell and thicken. He felt that as the cornea in the right eye had not deteriorated as much as the cornea in the left, by removing the cataract in the right eye very gently I would have some visual improvement without causing the cornea to decompensate. We discussed the benefits and risks of cataract surgery and Mr Flynn gave me an information leaflet on the procedure. We also discussed the option of not doing surgery. I was anxious to go ahead with the cataract surgery in the right eye as I was getting older and my eyesight was very definitely getting worse. Mr Flynn was supportive of my decision and I was relieved, as well as apprehensive, that things were moving forward at last. I was listed for cataract surgery in the right eye on the 18th December, 2019 at Bon Secours Hospital, College Road Cork.

I received correspondence from Mr Flynn's Eye Clinic informing me that I would be a day case patient, meaning that I would not be detained overnight in hospital. A local anaesthetic would be administered so I would be awake during the surgery. I was also reminded to bring the eyedrops which Mr Flynn had prescribed on my last appointment. I was requested to be at the Admissions Office, Bon Secours Hospital, Cork at 2.30pm on the 18th December 2019. The procedure itself would take about one hour, but that some waiting would be inevitable. I was told to expect to be in hospital for two to three hours for pre-operative and post-operative counselling and examination.

My wife, Sheila drove me to Cork for the surgery. I was very grateful for her company and her presence with me in the hospital before and after the surgery. I always refer to Sheila as one of the two rocks in my life. In all the years of our married life, she has given me rock solid support in good and bad times. I hope I have reciprocated in kind. My other rock, of course, is Austin Stacks GAA Club, Tralee, which is known locally as *The Rock*. It's a club for which I have had a lifelong affection since I first began playing juvenile football at the age of eight or nine.

Once I had signed in, I was escorted to the day ward where all the preliminary steps were carried out by the nursing staff. I was then wheeled up to the Operating Theatre where a local anaesthetic was administered. Mr Flynn and his support team then carried out the cataract surgery. I lost all track of time but I knew I was in the best of hands and Mr Flynn was very encouraging by addressing me from time to time with phrases like "all going very well, Billy." It was unusual to be awake while being operated on but I saw for myself - correction I heard for myself as my face, other than my right eye, was covered by a sterile drape - the excellent teamwork, care and professionalism with which the medical team approached the surgery. I could only admire and be grateful for the standard of medical practice in Ireland. After the procedure, a bandage was placed over my right eye for the first twenty-four hours after my surgery.

Sheila was waiting for me when I was returned to the ward. I felt very tired but I vaguely remember a nurse and Sheila taking about blood pressure and temperature and some other medical details. Sometime later, Mister Flynn dropped by to check on the eye and was very pleased with the outcome. Before checking out, I was given some day case follow up written instructions by the hospital.

1) You must be accompanied by a responsible adult

2) During the first 24 hours after your sedation/anaesthesia, ensure that someone stays in the house with you

3) During the first 24 hours after your sedation/anaesthesia, ensure you have access to a telephone

4) During the first 24 hours after your sedation/anaesthesia, do not drive, operate machinery, ride a bicycle, cook or take alcohol

5) Your short-term memory may be impaired for 48 hours after sedation/anaesthesia so you should not make any important business decisions or sign legal documents during this period.

Good advice indeed! I certainly had no intention of power washing the paths, cooking a meal or cycling down to the Pub for a few drinks to wash it down. Most of all, I was most definitely not going to sign any Last Will & Testament that was placed before me in the next 24 hours!

I had also studied the instructions and advice given to me by Mister Flynn.

AFTERCARE INSTRUCTIONS

First step is to remove the eye pad on the morning following cataract surgery. You may need to clean the eye because the drops and healing process can cause slight stickiness. You should clean your eyes before putting in your drops.

ADVICE ON CLEANING YOUR EYE

- Boil some water and allow it to cool

- Wash your hands

- Use a cotton bud dipped in the cooled boiled water to wipe across the eye lashes from the inner corner to the outer corner. Be careful not to press on the eye

- Repeat this using a clean tissue or cotton bud to remove any sticky deposits from your lid and lashes

- Dispose of the used tissues or cotton buds and wash your hands

- The white of the eye will appear red in patches. This is normal

AFTER SURGERY ADVICE

- Take the eye drops as per the prescription

- Wear the eye shield when sleeping during the first four nights after surgery to prevent pressure on the eye from a pillow or a hand while sleeping

- Do not rub your eyes after surgery

ADDITIONAL ADVICE

- For the first four weeks, face and hair washing must be done without getting water or shampoo in the eye. Wash hair backwards and perhaps, use cotton wool and cleanser for the face. Try not to get water or shampoo in the eyes in the shower

- Do not drive until your vision meets driving standard. This can take a few weeks and occasionally longer, especially if glasses are required. This will be discussed at your first follow-up appointment

- We strongly advise you not to travel abroad before your first post-operative review

- For the first week, avoid exercise in any case of injury or sweat running into the eyes. You may resume normal activities including golf, tennis, etc., after one week. Do not swim for four weeks after surgery.

Mister Flynn had already prescribed a course of eye drops, which I would begin at home after the cataract surgery. I was to take two different drops. The first was an antibiotic and the second was an anti-inflammatory. Now, it might seem like a simple task to place a drop into the eye, but when one is self-administering the drop, take my word for it, it can be hit or miss unless the aim is good. To help with the accuracy of the drop, Mister Flynn has developed a technique for instilling eyedrops. He refers to it as the *wrist-knuckle technique*, I found it to be very effective. It takes practice to make perfect as a dropper but, I assure you, I've had lots of practice during the past few years.

THE WRIST-KNUCKLE TECHNIQUE

1) Check the expiry date on your eye drop bottle and shake if required

2) Wash your hands before opening the bottle

3) Lie down or sit down and tilt your head back

4) Make a fist with one hand and use your knuckles to pull your lower eyelid downwards. Place your other hand with the eye drop bottle onto your knuckles

5) Look up and squeeze one drop into your lower eyelid, making sure the nozzle does not touch your eye, eyelashes or eyelid

6) Close your eye and press gently on the inner corner of your eye for 30 to 60 seconds to ensure the drop is fully absorbed

Christmas Day was just a week after the cataract surgery and I had been an enthusiastic participant in the Christmas Day swim at noon in Fenit for longer that I care to remember. There is something magical about lining up on the beach with the huge crowd of participants and joining in the rendition of Jingle Bells at five minutes to mid-day. Then counting down from ten second to noon and charging into the freezing sea. It's a long-standing tradition and whets the appetite for dinner. On my way home from Cork, I mentioned to Sheila that I might have to break my long sequence of Christmas Day swims. Sheila felt I should attend the swim only as a spectator but I knew that I'd find it very difficult to watch the swimmers enjoying the dip while I stood idly by on the shore-line. Eventually, after a great deal of discussion at home an acceptable compromise was reached. I didn't line up with the multitude of swimmers for the charge into the sea and the dive into the freezing water. I remained one step removed from the crowd and calmy strolled into the sea up to knee deep in the water. It really tested my willpower not to dive headlong into the sea but I accepted that it could not happen on this occasion. I had been given clear instructions by Mister Flynn which I was determined to follow. He had played his part by putting his expertise at my disposal. It was up to me to be patient and do the right thing. It wasn't the best Christmas swim I've ever had, but I did participate by stepping into the water and I really enjoyed the craic and the atmosphere that is unique to Fenit on Christmas Day.

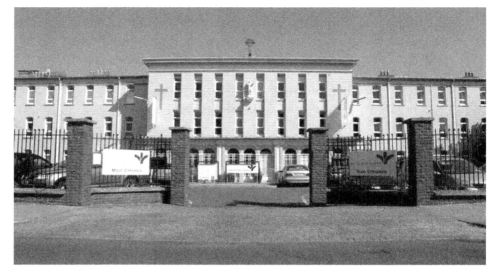

Bon Secours Hospital, College Road, Cork

CHAPTER ELEVEN

MISTER CHAIRMAN

In early December 2019, a strange turn of events resulted in me following an unexpected path for the following two years. Máiread Fernane, Chairperson of Austin Stacks GAA Club, who is a close personal friend of mine and for whom I have great respect and admiration, announced that she would be stepping down from the top position at the forthcoming Annual General Meeting. Máiread had given sterling service to the club down through the years. She had also served as Vice-Chairperson of the club and had made history by becoming the first female Chairperson of Austin Stacks. Her term in the chair had been very successful. Her pleasant personality, her organisational ability and management skills made her a very popular Chairperson. On the field, the club had been very successful. The club's senior team had already captured the 2019 Kerry Senior Club Football Championship, the premier competition for senior teams in the county. The team had also qualified for the semi-final of the County League, Division One. A unique double was now on the cards.

I was approached about taking over as Chairman. Initially, I was reluctant as I felt there were others in the club who were far more qualified for the job than myself. I was also conscious of the fact that I was suffering from Fuchs Dystrophy, which would necessitate a number of surgical procedures. It was very possible that my ability to act as Chairman might be compromised by any deterioration in my eyesight. I had been Secretary of the club some years early. I felt that I had done an efficient job and, I must admit, that the possibility of becoming Chairman of such a great club did appeal to me. I discussed the matter with my wife, Sheila, who gave me her unequivocal vote of confidence knowing how much The Rock meant to me. She also assured me, to my great relief, that she would be available to drive me to away games during my term of office. I realised that this was my opportunity to repay Austin Stacks for the values, ambitions and standards it had instilled in me since I was a young school boy attending CBS Primary School, Fairies Cross, Tralee back in the day.

I began to take soundings from people within the club whose opinions I valued. The feedback was very positive. When I was satisfied that I was the popular choice of club members, I began to take a serious look at the structures within the club and to prioritise my objectives. First of all, as I was well aware from my involvement in a number of clubs and organisations, any Chairman is far more effective if the Vice-Chairman is a reliable and wise confidant. It's vital for cohesion and unity within any organisation to have the first and second officers singing off the same hymn sheet. My choice was Éamonn O'Reilly, a man who had impressed me in a subcommittee we shared. I was delighted when Éamonn agreed to come on board and I was glad to have a man with his football brain by my side. Éamonn also had a distinguished reputation as a dynamic Chief Executive Officer of North East West Kerry Development Company. Éamonn deserves great credit for our achievement of the Holy Grail in 2021, but more about that later.

By the time of the 2019 Annual General Meeting at 10.30am on Sunday, 15th December 2019, our senior football team had qualified for the final of the Senior County League Division One against Rathmore. Whether by design or coincidence, the final was due to be played in Rathmore that very same afternoon. There was a great turn out at the AGM and the atmosphere was charged with giddy anticipation of new faces at the top table and the big game. I aimed to get my term up and running with a thoroughly researched address.

I began by wishing the Chairperson and members a Happy & Holy Christmas and Prosperity and Good Health in 2020. I expressed the hope that we would all get an early Christmas present in Rathmore on that afternoon with victory in the game against the home team.

"Thank you for electing me as your new Chairman for 2020," I continued. "It's a privilege to take on this position in the Austin Stacks Club, where my roots are deeply imbedded. It's a job I'm taking on after careful consideration and I'm certainly aware of the responsibility that it places on my shoulders.

Our great club is steeped in a century of history and I'm following in the footsteps of giants, beginning with Big Dan O Sullivan in 1917 and followed by twenty-nine distinguished Chairpersons, the last four being Ger Reidy, Aidan O'Connor, Liam Lynch and currently, Mairéad Fernane, a niece and goddaughter of Big Dan.

I will put time and effort into the position and I will engage with it to the best of my ability. My only agenda will be to do what's best for The Rock. I will be a Chairman for the entire club – gents, ladies and our valued young members. I only hope that I have the skills required to make a positive impact. If I'm to be an effective and progressive Chairman, I will need your goodwill and active support during the year. I'm confident that I'll get it in abundance.

I'm taking over as Chairman at a time when the Club is in rude health. We are very successful on and off the field. For more than a 100yrs, sometimes in very difficult circumstances, the Austin Stacks Club has fostered Gaelic games, Irish culture and Irish Republicanism.

For over 50yrs, we were homeless and nomadic. In 1971, Chairman Frank King and his Club Executive Committee purchased our new facilities in Connolly Park. We owe a huge debt of gratitude to that committee and the subsequent committees which developed the excellent facilities we now enjoy. We must never take for granted what we now have.

Now more than ever, we need members to step up to the plate to take on the various roles required to run an ambitious GAA Club. The Rock is famous on the field of play but it's also admired as a Club with sound structures, high standards, good organisation and willing workers.

As incoming Chairman, I'm adopting, with a slight modification, the motto of President John F Kennedy from his 1961 inauguration speech:

'Ask not what your Club can do for you - ask what you can do for your Club.'

So, today I am asking you, our members, to give everything to your club. Ask for nothing in return other than the satisfaction of being a valued member of one of the greatest GAA clubs in Ireland.

I am requesting supporters of The Rock, who don't pay the annual membership fee to dig deep and pay up for 2020. The more income the club generates, the better the service we can provide for our general membership, especially our young male and female members. Active and healthy involvement in Gaelic games from an early age is an ideal preparation for life. Our Juvenile Club under Chairman Tim McMahon and his dedicated team provides one of the finest under-age structures in the country. Our Ladies Club, chaired by Noreen Power, continues to go from strength to strength. Your membership fee will help to sustain that wonderful work.

I'd like to thank the members of the 2019 Executive Committee for your outstanding work during the year. I'm extremely grateful to those of you who are staying on in 2020. I will be availing of your experience, advice, wisdom and guidance during the year. My gratitude to all who serve on subcommittees, prepare our teams, look after our pitches, raise funds and who help out in any way. You are the beating heart of the Club.

To our outgoing Chairperson, I'd like to say: Mairéad, you have earned your place alongside Big Dan in the glorious history of The Rock Club. You have the distinction of being the first female Chairperson of our club. That honour is yours forever. You have been an outstanding Chairperson and Vice-Chairperson of Austin Stacks. Mairéad, in your courteous and gracious style, you have done The Rock some service. I will be calling on you, from time to time, to do some more!

Finally, I'd like to extend seasonal greetings to Rockies at home and abroad. I cordially invite Rock people, who are living away from home to be part of our club in 2020. Keep in touch through our club web site, the print media and social media. Better still, become a member of the club for 2020. Once a Rockie, always a Rockie!"

The icing on the cake was our thrilling victory over a gallant Rathmore team at Rathmore later on in the day. Our supporters turned out in large numbers and their encouragement was greatly appreciated by the team and myself. The game was very exciting and played in a fine sporting manner by both teams. By full time, the sides couldn't be separated. Even extra time failed to produce a result. So, it all came down to penalty kicks and who else but Kieran Donaghy stepped up to the plate to take the decisive penalty. Cool as a breeze Star slotted the ball into the back of the net to complete the double of Club Championship and League Championship for Austin Stacks. Not many Chairmen have been privileged to be elected and to have his club team win a prestigious title on the same day!

I could take little credit for the wonderful double. Credit where credit is due to the focussed stewardship of my predecessor, Mairéad Fernane. But such is the character of the lady that Mairéad shared the success with me. We stood for a photograph together and we went to the dressing room to congratulate our victorious team. I was due for cataract surgery in Cork three days later on the 18th December 2019. It never entered my mind on that super Sunday as I was the happiest person in Kerry! It was a very special day.

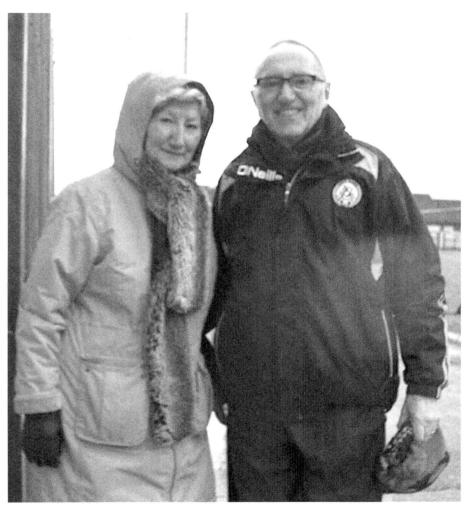

Mairéad Fernane and Billy Ryle at the Kerry Senior Football League, Division One Final in Rathmore on the 15th December 2019

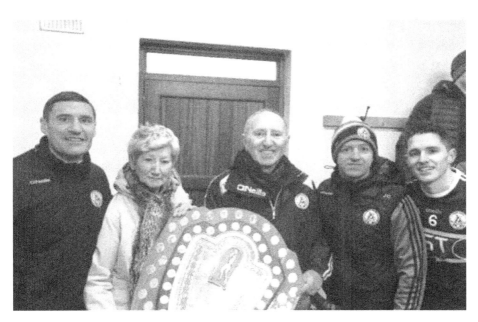

From left, Wayne Quillinan, Mairéad Fernane, Billy Ryle, Jonathan Conway and Ronan Shanahan at the Kerry Senior Football League, Division One Final in Rathmore on the 15th December 2019

CHAPTER TWELVE

CATARACT SURGERY SUCCESS

Subsequent to my procedure in December 2019, an appointment was arranged for me to see Mr Flynn at The Elysian on 10th January 2020. By that stage I was reaping the benefit of the cataract surgery in my right eye. The vision in that eye had certainly improved and the haze, which I still had in the left eye, had considerably lessened in the right eye. I was delighted that the surgery had helped to improve my vision.

The letter with the appointment details always contained invaluable information about preparing for the appointment and recommendations in relation to driving to and from the appointment. The letter made it clear that the examination of the eye at the appointment would possibly involve eyedrops to dilate the pupils. The drops blur vision temporarily, lasting between four to six hours, so the letter strongly advised a patient not to drive to or from the consultation.

I had already resolved not to do any long-distance driving until I had completed my eye treatment, which would involve two cataract surgeries and two corneal transplants of donor organs. From listening to Mr Flynn, I came to appreciate that the corneal transplant surgery was a more delicate operation than the cataract surgery and I could sense his reluctance to go ahead with it until it was absolutely necessary. At this stage, I implicitly trusted his judgement and I was in there for the long haul, whatever length of time it took. I had accepted that I would be making regular trips to Cork over the next few years. I was up for it and fully prepared to go with the flow. In addition, at the end of each appointment with Mr Flynn, I was given a date for the next appointment. Knowing when next I had to be in Cork gave me plenty of time to organise my schedule.

When my wife Sheila was free, she drove me to Cork for my appointment. I really enjoyed her company and her uncanny knack of keeping my spirits up. I have always had a steely resilience in coping with the ups and downs of life but Sheila's optimism and encouragement was very uplifting. Her motivational talks often brought Rudyard Kipling's famous poem, *IF* to my mind, a few lines of which I quote below.

"If you can keep your head when all about you
Are losing theirs and blaming it on you,
If you can wait and not be tired by waiting,
If you can meet with Triumph and Disaster
And treat those two impostors just the same;
If you can fill the unforgiving minute
With sixty seconds' worth of distance run,
Yours is the Earth and everything that's in it,
And—which is more—you'll be a Man, my son!"

I had a tendency to mentally add a few inadequate lines of my own to the poem to express my feelings about my wife.

"If you have the love of a good and loyal woman
Who steadfastly stands by your side in all adversity
If you know you will never have to walk alone
Then you are a very lucky Man, my son!"

(With profound apologies to Kipling)

If anything, our regular trips to Cork brought Sheila and I even closer. We had time to chat about the many blessings that came our way during forty-two years of married life. We laughed at the many adventures we shared with our growing up children Kevin, Gráinne and Brian. We reminisced about their school days. We recalled some of the wonderful celebrations we had together - birthdays, Sacraments, exam successes, college graduations, and so on. We wondered how Aisling would have turned out if she had been given a life to live. We shed a tear in her memory. And, of course, we marvelled at the great joy our beloved grandchildren Kate, Liam, Max and Jack had brought into our lives. We have so much to be grateful for.

On the occasions that Sheila was unable to drive me to Cork, I usually took the 9am train from Tralee to Cork. It was lovely to sit back and relax. Sometimes, I just enjoyed the view out through the window. Sometimes I'd read a book but, most of all, I'd enjoy chatting with other travellers. Having a natural interest in people and their myriad of stories, I was fascinated by what they had to say and where they were going. I met people heading off on holidays, people travelling to Dublin or Cork for a day out and people who, like myself, had a medical appointment. If a train could talk, it would have a great story to tell about its eclectic mix of travellers of all ages on journeys to only God knows where.

Another advantage of travelling by train is the proximity of Kent Railway Station in Cork, to The Elysian. I could walk it comfortably in seven or eight minutes. As my appointment was usually scheduled for 12 noon, 12.15pm or 12.30pm, I was left with plenty of time afterwards for a bite of lunch before catching the 2.25pm train to Tralee where I could meet up with Sheila around 5pm. One big advantage of driving to Cork was that, after the appointment with Mr Flynn, we weren't tied to any timetable. The rest of the day was our own. Now that all our chicks had flown the nest, we were at liberty to head into town, Mahon, Blackpool or Wilton for some shopping and lunch or as they say in Cork, to shoot the breeze down Pana. In Kerry speak that translates to enjoying a leisurely stroll along Patrick Street.

At the appointment of 10th January 2020, Mr Flynn gave my eyes a thorough examination. He was pleased that my right eye was settling down after the cataract surgery and that the procedure had improved my vision in that eye. In a follow up letter to Dr O'Regan, which was courtesy copied to me, Mister Flynn described my eye problems as Fuchs endothelial dystrophy in both eyes, cataract in the left eye and pseudophakic - IOL in the bag. While that is professional Doctor to Doctor terminology, I understood it to mean that I would need cataract surgery in the left eye and a corneal transplant of donor organs in both eyes. I was delighted when Mr Flynn said that the right eye was settling well after the December 2019 surgery and that he was pleased with the level of improvement in my vision. I was called back again for further post-operative consultations on the 21st February 2020 and the 28th February 2020, when the feedback from Mr Flynn gave me a great lift,

It was now over two months since I had the right eye cataract surgery. Mr Flynn said that the cornea in my right eye remained slightly thicker than before the cataract surgery but that it was optically clear. Now that my vision had improved the time had come to get new glasses for optimal vision. Mr Flynn felt that the corneal thickening was not bad enough to warrant surgery and he was hopeful that it would improve over the next few months. He advised me to hold off surgery on the left eye until we saw the final result of the right eye with glasses. He said he would see me again in about three months and his Practice Co-Ordinator confirmed an appointment for me at 12.15pm on the 29th May 2020.

CHAPTER THIRTEEN

BUSY DIARY

My term as Austin Stacks Chairman got off to a wonderful start and within a month, I had finalised the members of the Club Executive, set up the appropriate subcommittees and had mentors in place for all of our teams. Everybody was looking forward to our training routine and football games which would begin as soon as the weather improved. I was very conscious of the voracious appetite for success that existed throughout the club. Our juvenile structure was very well organised and regularly won titles in all grades. We fielded three senior teams in various competitions and I was very anxious for all of them to lift silverware. The three premier competitions which were available to our Senior A team were Kerry Senior League Division One, Kerry Senior Club Football Championship and Kerry Senior Football Championship. We had won the first two competitions in 2019 but the blue riband County Senior Football Championship had eluded Austin Stacks since our last success in 2014. I was determined to win that prestigious trophy during my term. The problem was that the East Kerry Divisional team were dominant in Kerry. The unmarkable David Clifford was the main man on that team but it was a very strong side throughout the field. It would take some performance by our Austin Stacks team to get the better of East Kerry, but it was possible. From the beginning luck was on my side. Brendan and Paul O'Sullivan from Valentia Island relocated to Tralee for employment and decided to throw in their lot with Austin Stacks. Brendan and Paul slotted in to our squad like a hand in a glove. They were both talented footballers who considerably strengthened our team. They had a hunger for success and were prepared to train hard to achieve it. In addition, both of them were very likeable and unassuming young men.

The Chairman's role also involved representing the club at various functions, the first of which was the annual dinner of Connolly Park

Residents Association on Sunday, 19th January 2020. Sheila and I were made very welcome and enjoyed a beautiful meal. I said a few words and treated the attendance to a few songs. I enjoy an occasional sing song but I'm only in the halfpenny place when compared to my late second cousin, Dusty Springfield, whose mother was Kay Ryle from Tralee. Our playing pitches are known as Connolly Park alongside a residential estate, also called Connolly Park. Austin Stacks maintains a very close cordial working relationship with the residents who are very generous in helping out with our activities. For example, the dinner I mentioned above is held annually in our club function room. Connolly Park Residents Association, for example, assists us with parking arrangements for and stewarding of games.

On the following evening Monday, 20th January, 2020 I hosted a press night to announce details of our upcoming victory social. We felt it was important to treat our supporters to a good night out to celebrate our many successes on the field in 2019. I gave a presentation at the press night which was held in our Club facilities in Connolly Park. I began by welcoming the members of the media, Ms Michelle King, Director of Sales & Marketing at the Rose Hotel, Tralee, members, supporters and friends of the Austin Stack Hurling & Football Club to the press briefing. I said that I was delighted to announce that the Austin Stack GAA Club would be hosting 'The Rock & Rose Victory Social' at the Rose Hotel, Dan Spring Road, Tralee on Saturday, 22nd February 2020 to celebrate six outstanding trophy successes in 2019.

"Our senior football team under the management team of Wayne Quillinan, Eoin Colgan, Jonathan Conway, John O Sullivan, Tommy Naughton and Damien Ryall won the Kerry Senior Club Championship – defeating Dr Crokes in the final. Then on Sunday, 15th December 2019 in a wet and windy Rathmore, history was made when our gallant senior team completed a unique double by winning the final of the Senior County League, Division One in the most dramatic fashion. With the teams – Stacks and Rathmore - still level at 1-10 each after normal time and extra time had been played, a penalty shoot-out was used for the first time in Kerry to decide the title. In a nerve-wracking climax,

Stacks took the Senior League Division One title by scoring four penalties to Rathmore's three – the decisive fourth penalty being calmly dispatched to the back of the Rathmore net by our *Star* himself, Kieran Donaghy.

Our senior team also did the double in Tralee District Board competitions by winning both the District League Final against Ballymacelligott and the District Championship Final against John Mitchels.

Our C team, affectionally known as Charlie's Angels, in memory of the late Charlie Healy also achieved a double success. Under the management of Aidan O Connor, Ricky Moloney, John Joe Sugrue, Tommy O Connor, Daniel Bohan, Ger Mannix and Ciaran McCabe they won both the County Junior League and the County Junior Championship, bringing the Barrett Cup back to the Rock.

Our Senior B team managed by Paddy Barry, Eamonn O Reilly and Kieran Kelliher, played in Division Five of the County League. Although they didn't win silverware, they reached the final of their championship for the Molyneaux Cup, narrowly losing out to Dr Crokes. The team also finished joint fourth in the league, just missing out on a promotion playoff. As many of these stars of the future were needed during the year for Senior A team duty, they will be entitled to medals at the Social.

I'd also like to mention that Austin Stacks is Tralee's largest Ladies Club, catering for girls from U-6 to senior. Our Senior Ladies last won the County Intermediate Championship in 2017 and are on the cusp of another major success. In 2019, the club had no less than nine players involved with Kerry Teams. I am very grateful to Chairperson Noreen Power and her dedicated team officials for their superb work in fostering ladies' football in The Rock.

The commitment, time and effort that our teams and management have put into the past season was incredible. These very dedicated groups deserved success on the playing field. I am very grateful for all that they do to bring success to The Rock.

Of course, success is hard won and must be celebrated as life moves on very quickly. For that reason, I am calling for a huge turn-out of Rockies and their friends at the Rock & Rose Victory Social at the Rose Hotel on Saturday, 22nd February 2020. Come along and pay tribute to our teams and officials. I can assure you that Siobhán Power, Chairperson of our Social & Cultural Subcommittee and her team are organising a great night of celebration in a convivial atmosphere, beginning with a champagne reception at 7.30pm and followed by a wonderful meal. After the medal presentation, the young and the young at heart can dance the night away to the music of Heart & Soul and DJ Francie Breen.

A highlight of the night will be the announcement of Club Lady of the Year 2019 and Club Man of the Year 2019. That will be a difficult task for the judges but it will remain a closely guarded secret until the night. Social tickets at €35 each will be on sale this weekend from, Siobhán Power, Lorraine Scanlon and Mary Mc Quinn. The girls will also sell tickets at the club on a number of nights. All details will be posted on our social media outlets and our club notes," I continued.

I was delighted to say a few words to the parents and young players who attended our Juvenile Club registration evening on Wed, 5th February 2020. I explained that Austin Stacks was a large club, a famous club and a club which was highly regarded for its on-field successes. The club was also highly respected for its promotion of high standards, best behaviour and sportsmanship. I pointed out that the club is governed by an Executive Committee which is elected at our Annual General Meeting and has representatives from all branches of our club.

"The Club Executive" I said, "is made up of very skilled and committed people and it is my privilege to be Chairman of such a wonderful club. The club has four main arteries – senior, juvenile, ladies and hurling – all of which are flourishing except for hurling which I hope to address as the year progresses.

Our Juvenile Club is thriving under Chairman Tim McMahon, Secretary Mike Lynch, Treasurer Eileen Nagle and their very dedicated committee and team officials. Our Juvenile Club from our U-6, U-8 and U-10 Academy right up the U-16 level is the jewel in the crown of our club. Our juvenile teams are consistently winners in their competitions.

Our Juvenile Club provides a regular flow of players for our U-18, U-21 and Senior teams. Many of our players go on to represent Kerry at all levels right up to senior level. I'd like to mention that we have nine players on the Tralee CBS team which has qualified for the Munster Colleges Senior Football final. Tim Mc Mahon is the Manager of The Green team.

Our club philosophy is to develop personal skills such as loyalty, self-discipline, work-ethic, ambition, initiative, team-work and determination in our young players as well as football skills - kicking, fetching, passing, blocking, marking and so on.

Our Juvenile Club has top class high calibre coaches at all levels. Our team mentors encourage and support our young players in a safe environment and ensure that they all get playing time on the pitch. Our club is a happy club where our young members enjoy themselves, have fun, build character and make long lasting friendships.

Our Club Executive is determined that all of our players from senior level to U-6 will always have the best training facilities, gear, equipment and support structures. Cost is always the elephant in the room!

So, I'd like to ask those of you who are not club members to join the club. A variety of memberships is available to suit all circumstances. Your membership will enable us to provide a better service. Bernie Mannix, our club Registrar will give you full details of club membership and our weekly Lotto, which is a vital source of income for us.

We hold a number of fund-raising events during the year. Please support them in whatever way you can. We would also appreciate your support in organising the events and helping out on the day.

Our Rock & Rose Victory Social, to celebrate winning six senior trophies in 2019, goes ahead at The Rose Hotel on Saturday, 22nd February 2020. It will be a great night of celebration. Tickets at €35 each will be on sale at the club between 8pm & 9pm on Friday night. I would love to see you at the Social.

Our juvenile members will enjoy the football during the year. They will benefit not just as footballers but also as individuals from their involvement with The Rock. Thank you for registering with Austin Stacks and becoming a valued part of our great club."

The Registration night was very successful and it was very refreshing to chat informally with the large cohort of parents who were present. I was overwhelmed by the goodwill they felt for the club and how excited they were about the new season ahead. I felt confident that a large number of the parents present would, at some stage, take an active role in the club's activities. Nights like this were very a very important exercise in public relations for the club. Tim McMahon and his team had done a great job in organising it and I was certain that the experience that the young players would have in the next few months would live up to what was promised on the night.

Speaking about young people, Mercy Primary School, Balloonagh backs on to our playing pitches in Connolly Park. Many of the young people who attend Balloonagh school are members of our Juvenile Club. We have always enjoyed a warm mutual relationship which is beneficial to both school and club. For example, the school authorities have free use of our pitches when they require them. If we ever need to talk to the children about enrolling with Austin Stacks, we are always made most welcome. I, myself, am a past pupil of Balloonagh school and I have always had a great affinity with the school and some lovely memories of the wonderful time I spent there. When I took over as Chairman of Austin Stacks, the school authorities already had a major building extension in progress. In order to fundraise for the new building, the school decided to hold a Valentine's Ball on Friday 14th February 2020 at Ballygarry House Hotel in Ballyseedy, Tralee. Each table, which sat ten people, would cost €1,000. I was anxious to support the event because of my affection for the school and to further cement the cordial working relationship between school and club. I had little or no difficulty in getting eight other club members to join Sheila and I at what was a wonderful event. As dress was formal, it gave me an opportunity to don my black dress suit with bow tie and Sheila to dress for the occasion as ladies like to do. She looked stunning on the night and we both had a very enjoyable evening.

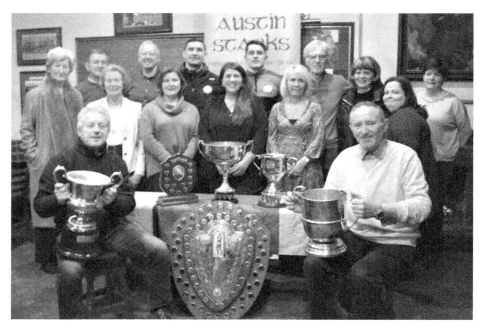

At the Press Conference on the 20th January 2020 to announce detail of 'The Rock & Rose Victory Social' were
Front Row: L/r Éamonn O'Reilly, Vice-Chairman and Billy Ryle, Chairman
Second Row: L/r Mairéad Fernane, Carmel Quilter O'Neill, Elma Nix, Mary McQuinn, Lorraine Scanlon and Siobhán Power
Back Row: L/r Nial Shanahan, Colm Mangan, Wayne Quillinan, Ronan Shanahan, Aidan O'Connor, Michelle King and Anne Marie Healy

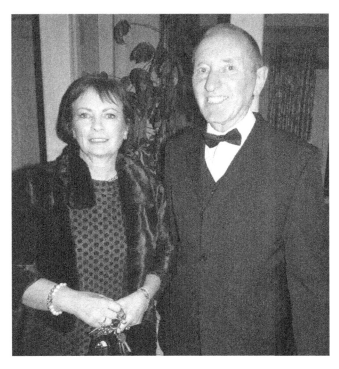

Billy & Sheila Ryle attended the Balloonagh Primary School's Valentine Day Fundraising Ball at Ballygarry Hotel, Tralee on the 14th February 2020   Photo courtesy of Carol Anne O'Donoghue

CHAPTER FOURTEEN

ROCK & ROSE VICTORY SOCIAL

Just about a week later on Saturday 22nd February 2020, the Austin Stacks Victory Social went ahead at The Rose Hotel, Tralee. The atmosphere was electric from early evening as a huge crowd gathered in the Hotel Foyer for a champagne reception. That was followed by a beautiful meal in the main Reception Hall. The presentation of medals and special awards brought the house down. There was constant cheering and revelry as the players came up to receive their medals from me. The names of the winners of the special awards were kept under lock and key until they were announced on the night and greeted with huge acclaim.

I had put a great deal of preparation into my speech, which was intended to acknowledge what had been achieved in 2019 and to set out our stall for more success in 2020. I was conscious also that the remains of the club's oldest member, Séan Murphy had been returned earlier in the day to his native Carlow for burial. I was also in a position to announce our new generous sponsorship deal with The Brogue Inn Bar & Restaurant, Rock Street and I was going to avail of the opportunity to make a pitch for sponsors for our other teams. I was about to earn my dinner!

"Fr. Padraig Walsh, Fr Seán Hanafin, Brendan Dowling, President of Austin Stacks, Eamonn Whelan, Vice-Chairman, Kerry County Board GAA, invited Guests, Ladies & Gentlemen," I began, "welcome to The Rock & Rose Victory Social, celebrating six outstanding trophy successes in 2019, including the Kerry Senior Club Championship and the County Senior League, Division One.

As you know, Séan Murphy, the oldest member of our Club, in his 99th year, passed away on Tuesday. We accompanied his remains to the Church of Our Lady & St Brendan last evening. After his Requiem Mass early today, his remains were returned to his native Carlow for burial. Séan was introduced to The Rock by Kevin Barry in the late

'60's, when Séan first arrived in Tralee. He served the club as a football & hurling selector. He was our County Board delegate and served as Vice-Chairman. Séan was a Trustee of the Club until the time of his death.

By sheer coincidence, last Thursday we transferred the final payment of €5,000 for our second pitch, The Nuns' Field to the Diocesan Trust. Austin Stacks now owns every single blade of grass on The Nuns' Field thanks to Seán, his great friend Tadgh McMahon, John Lynch, Aidan O Connor, Canice Walsh and their contemporaries, who were brave enough to take the risk when the opportunity presented itself. Seán would want us to celebrate tonight and we will do that. So, on behalf of the Austin Stack Club, I will bid farewell to Seán.

Slán leat Seán, a chara. Go ndeanfaidh Dia trocaire ar d'anam uasal agus go mbeidh leaba agat i measc na naomh.

My motto as Chairman of this great club is adopted, with a slight modification, from John F Kennedy's inauguration speech as President of the USA: *"Ask not what your Club can do for you - ask what you can do for your Club."* And my God, our senior teams gave everything they had to the club during a remarkable year. The dedication shown by our teams during the past season was remarkable.

Our senior team, managed by Wayne Quillinan, Eoin Colgan, Jonathan Conway, John O Sullivan, Tommy Naughton,
Our senior B team managed by Paddy Barry, Eamonn O Reilly and Kieran Kelliher
and
Our senior C team managed by Aidan O Connor, Ricky Moloney, John Joe Sugrue, Tommy O Connor, Daniel Bohan, Ger Mannix and Ciaran McCabe thoroughly deserved their successes on the playing field. The club is very grateful to the players and management teams for what they achieved last year. Not only did the players give everything on the playing field, but they did so with the high standards, exemplary behaviour and sportsmanship for which Austin Stacks is renowned. Management and players, you are a credit to our club and we are very

proud of each and every one of you. Congratulations on your success in 2019 and best wishes for the year ahead.

Our Ladies' Club is going from strength to strength under Chairperson Noreen Power and her dedicated team. They are doing superb work in fostering ladies' football in The Rock and I'm confident that 2020 will be a big year for our ladies' teams.

Our Juvenile Club is thriving under Chairman Tim McMahon and his dedicated officials. Our Juvenile Club is the jewel in the crown of The Rock, consistently winning competitions in all age groups and providing a regular flow of players for our minor, U21 and senior teams. The future of the Rock is in good hands.

I'd like to thank Colin Teahan and his company, PST Sport for being our main sponsor for the past eight years. The Club has great affection for Colin, who was not only a very generous sponsor but also a genuine supporter.

I'm delighted to announce this evening that Kirby's Brogue Inn Bar & Restaurant, Rock Street, Tralee will be our main club sponsors for the next three years. We'll have a formal launch in due course. We are delighted to link up with a Rock St business with strong connections to our club. I'd like to thank Kevin & Fiona Cotter for their generous financial backing. Our senior players will do their very best to repay them with silverware.

Our under-age team sponsorship proposal ranging from minor level down to our academy is now available. We have a very attractive package on offer at affordable cost. We are ready and willing to discuss a sponsorship agreement with any interested companies and businesses.

My sincere thanks to The Rose Hotel for hosting tonight's Social and for decking out the venue in our black and amber colours. The advice and assistance of the Hotel staff, especially Michelle King & Madeline Doyle was greatly appreciated. I know that the Hotel has a beautiful meal prepared for all of us.

I would like to thank Timmy Sheehan for being our Master of Ceremonies tonight. Timmy is the best at everything he does. We were in school together back in the day. From an early age, it was very obvious that Timmy was a classy footballer with a great career ahead of him. As a commentator and sports writer he is out on his own.

I want to thank our Club Executive Committee for enthusiastically backing tonight's Social and being very supportive during the past few weeks. Eamonn O'Reilly, Bernie Mannix, Ricky Maloney, Elma Nix and Martin Collins, in particular, together with Wayne Quillinan made very telling contributions.

But credit where credit is due. For the most part, the Social was organised by the energetic Siobhán Power, Chairperson of our Social and Cultural Subcommittee and her wonderful team. Nothing was left to chance. No task was too big or too small. No detail went unchecked. No phone call, text or email went unanswered. So, Siobhán, Mary, Lorraine, Noreen and company, a sincere thank you for organising this beautiful night out for the Rockies, our guests and our friends. Enjoy the function everybody."

Everybody was in great form for the presentation of medals and awards after the meal. Timmy Sheehan was magnificent in his introduction of the players. He had an anecdote to relay about each and every one of them. He had us all mesmerised by the power of his oratory and his endless depth of knowledge. I was so happy that he agreed to take the microphone for this special occasion. No one else could have done it better.

Timmy opened the medal presentation after dessert had been served and I had the honour of making the presentations, beginning with Senior A team, which was followed by the Senior C team. The announcement of Club Lady and Gent of the year to two very deserving winners, was greeted with huge acclaim. The citations from the judging panel were read out by Timmy. I include them below as well as the other deserving award winners.

Club Lady of the Year – Carmel Quilter O Neill

This club officer is a whirlwind of energy and the first to put her hand up to help with every club event. She is a passionate supporter who loves nothing better than following our teams. She is a club favourite of members young & old. Her dedication to Austin Stacks is best reflected in her simply amazing fundraising abilities. Some sing for their supper but this lady would, and has, sang and danced for a lotto ticket sale. The winner of the 2019 Club Lady of the year award is Carmel Quilter O Neill.

Club Man of the Year – Noel O Connell

No matter what's happening on any given day in Austin Stacks you can guarantee this man has had a hand in it. That has been the case for more years than we can remember. We speak for all players, team managers & club officers when we say that the club simply couldn't function without him. Obliging, reliable and a friend to all. For fixtures, help, advice & emergency 999 calls he's our go to man every time. The recipient of the 2019 Club Man of the year award is Noel O Connell.

- Senior Lady player of the Year   Jemma O Connell
- Senior C Team Player of the Year   David Courtney
- Senior B Team Player of the Year   Paul Galvin
- Senior A Team Player of the Year   Joe O Connor

There was great interest in the last two awards of the evening, best dressed lady and best dressed gent, as all of us like a bit of style and fashion. It must have been a hard call to make as the men were dressed handsomely and the ladies were at their stylish best. The deserving winners on the night were Breda O'Callaghan and Jack Morgan. After the formalities the dancing and merriment went on into the early hours of Sunday morning. All in all, it was a fabulous celebration.

Just to prove that life can quickly change from being a bed of roses to a vale of tears, I was deeply shocked when Timmy Sheehan died suddenly on the 3rd March 2020, just ten days after the Rock and Rose Victory Social. The Austin Stacks GAA Club, Tralee went into mourning following the sudden death of a dear friend and club colleague. The Club was shattered by the sudden and untimely loss of a former great player, coach, sports writer and commentator. It was very difficult to come to terms with the fact that Timmy would no longer be with us on the side line, pen and notebook in hand. His sport's column in The Kerryman newspaper would no longer be written. His march reports would no longer be heard on Radio Kerry. His expertise as a Master of Ceremonies would no longer be available. The Rock Club would sorely miss one it's most loyal sons.

I was very grateful to club members for the wonderful support, collectively and individually, they gave to the Sheehan family during that very difficult week. The massive turn out for the guard of honour which accompanied Timmy's remains to the Church of Our Lady and St. Brendan on the Friday night was one of our biggest ever. Despite torrential rain on Saturday afternoon, the large guard of honour escorting Timmy's remains for burial in Rath Cemetery was indicative of the affection that club members had for Timmy.

Austin Stack's Club PRO, Martin Collins, who was a close personal friend of Timmy delivered a memorable oration at Timmy's graveside, which was a glowing tribute to a life well lived. No one could have done it better than Martin and I am honoured to include it in this book.

Oration by Martin Collins, PRO Austin Stacks GAA Club, Tralee at the grave of Timmy Sheehan at Rath Cemetery, Tralee, Co. Kerry, on Saturday, 7th March 2020

"There was sorrow and disbelief throughout the county and beyond last week when news broke of the sudden death of Timmy Sheehan. Two days before his passing he was reporting for Radio Kerry on the Kerry/Antrim Senior Hurling National League game in Austin Stack Park.

After coming up through the Juvenile ranks of the 1960s, Timmy's first success at adult level came in 1967, when Stacks won the Kerry minor hurling championship. Timmy's midfield partner in that final was none other than Dick Spring. He then went on to have a glittering career at senior level – going on to win four Senior Football County Championship medals in 1973, 1975, 1976 and 1979. In between he won a Munster and an All-Ireland Club Senior Football Championship medal during the 1976/77 season. He also won five County League titles during this period and captained the team in 1974 – the year they won their second League title.

When his Senior days were over, he lined out with the Junior teams and was a member of the C team when they won their first Barrett Cup Final in 1986. Afterwards he was an outstanding coach and manager of many teams at both Junior and Senior levels down the years, including a very good Senior Hurling team which the Club had in the late 1980s-early 1990s. His son Billy was also an outstanding Club player and had a brilliant career with the Laois Senior Footballers from 2004 right up to 2016. Timmy continued his involvement with Club affairs right up to the end. Just ten days before he died, he brilliantly did the master of ceremonies at the Club's Annual Social when the Senior A and Senior C Team players were presented with their winners' medals after such a successful season.

In addition to his Club work, he was also a brilliant sports writer/ commentator with the local Kerryman Newspaper and Radio Kerry. His knowledge of most sports was second to none. Apart from GAA matters he excelled in Basketball and Soccer in particular and he was so pleased to see his beloved Liverpool moving close to winning the Premiership after a 30yr gap. A huge guard of honour of former and current players accompanied the cortege to Our Lady and St. Brendan's Church on last Friday's night and again to Rath Cemetery on Saturday afternoon.

We extend sincere sympathy to Timmy's wife, Anne; his daughter, Lorraine, his son Billy, his daughter in law Marie, his three grandsons – Timmy, Billy & Davie, and to all his extended family and friends. Ní bheidh a leithéid ann arís."

I was very thankful to our two senior teams who played so well at home in Connolly Park on the Sunday after Timmy's death in County League games that were dedicated to his memory. The respectful observation of the minute's silence by the players, mentors and the large attendance at the games was appreciated. It was the first time in many years that Timmy wasn't present with pen and note book at the ready. It was a difficult and sad week for The Rock, but I felt very proud to be Chairman of Austin Stacks, a club which showed fortitude and resilience in the loss of a noble member.

Shortly after Timmy's death, just when our season was up and running and the club was a hive of activity, the deadly virus from the Orient invaded our shores. It broke our hearts to have to lock the gates and to bring activities in Connolly Park to an abrupt halt. But it was the right thing to do and as an integral part of the GAA family we had no hesitation in complying with the directives from Croke Park. The World Health Organisation's categorisation of the coronavirus outbreak as a pandemic presented all of us with a serious challenge. The Austin Stack Club faced that challenge in a united and determined manner. We did so by proactively complying with the Government's national public health guidelines.

It was a particularly difficult time for our players, from the youngest to the oldest, who were denied the joy of training and the thrill of competing on the playing field. The best laid plans and timelines of our coaching staff were thrown into disarray. Year planning, administration and organisation by our Club officers and committees had to be revisited. Social activity in the Bar, fitness activity in the Gym and activity on the playing fields all came to a standstill.

The important thing is that every member of our club rose to the challenge and did what was necessary to rid us of the deadly Covid-19 virus. As well as that, the Austin Stacks GAA Club Community Response initiated by our senior players to lend a helping hand to those in need, filled me with pride in our great club.

I was thankful to our members for their patience, solidarity, cooperation, generosity of spirit, compassion and wholehearted support for The Rock's contribution to the national campaign to rid Ireland of the evil invader. Their actions helped our Club and the entire country to come safely through the worst of times.

From the beginning, I encouraged all of our club members to comply with the public health guidelines. I appealed to them to stay safe and well until we could once again do what we do best - indulge our passion for Gaelic games in our wonderful club. But for the foreseeable future the Covid-19 Virus had the country in its grip and our club was in complete lock down.

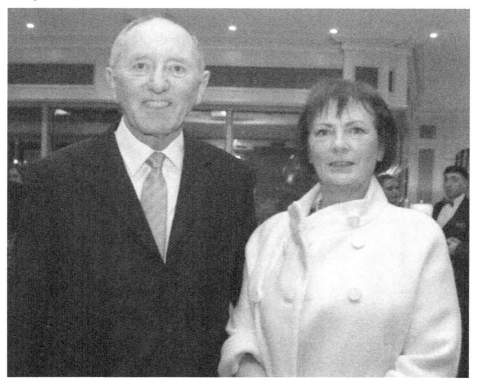

Billy & Sheila Ryle attended the Rock & Rose Victory Social at the Rose Hotel Tralee on 22nd February 2020
Photo courtesy of Dermot Crean

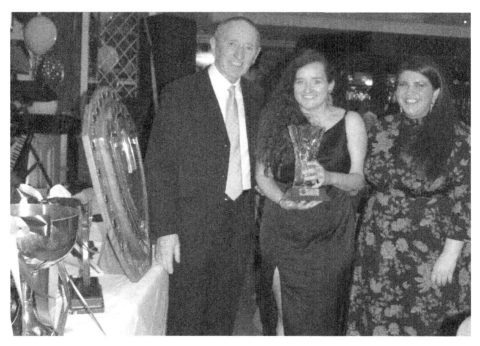

Gemma O'Connell, centre, lady player of the year at the Rock & Rose Victory Social with Billy Ryle and Mary McQuinn at the Rose Hotel Tralee on 22nd February 2020

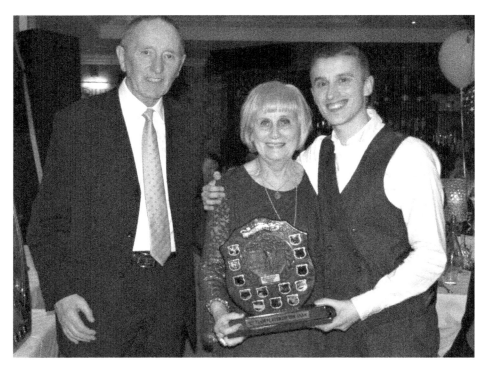

David Courtney, Senior C player of the year, on right, at the Rock & Rose Victory Social with Billy Ryle and Ena Healy at the Rose Hotel Tralee on 22nd February 2020

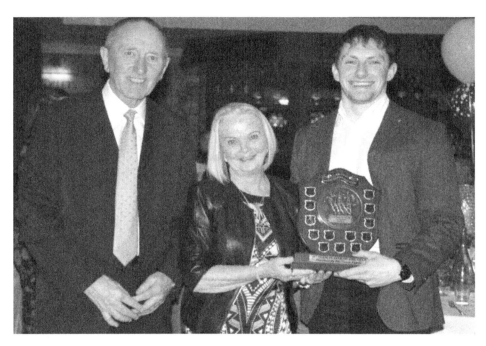

Paul Galvin, on right, Senior B player of the year at the Rock & Rose Victory Social with Billy Ryle and Noreen Power at the Rose Hotel Tralee on 22nd February 2020

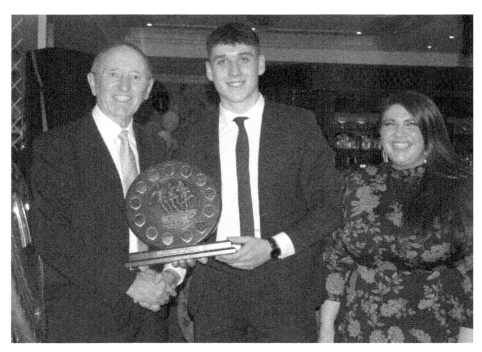

Joe O'Connor, centre, Senior A player of the year at the Rock & Rose Victory Social with Billy Ryle and Mary McQuinn at the Rose Hotel Tralee on 22nd February 2020

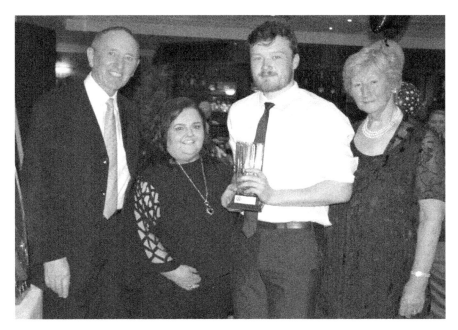

Ciarán O Connell, second right, accepts the Club man of the year award, on behalf of his father Noel, from Billy Ryle, Siobhán Power and Mairéad Fernane at the Rock & Rose Victory Social at the Rose Hotel Tralee on 22nd February 2020

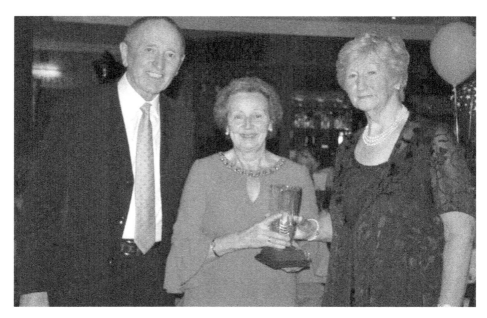

Carmel Quilter O'Neill, centre, accepts the Club lady of the year award from Mairéad Fernane and Billy Ryle at the Rock & Rose Victory Social at the Rose Hotel Tralee on 22nd February 2020

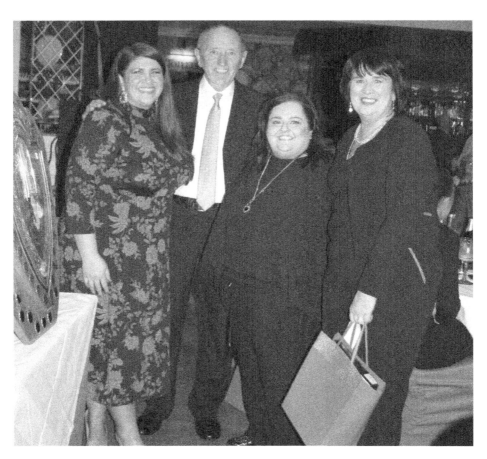

Breda O Callaghan, on right, best dressed lady at the Rock & Rose Victory Social at the Rose Hotel Tralee on 22nd February 2020 is pictured with Mary McQuinn, Billy Ryle and Siobhán Power

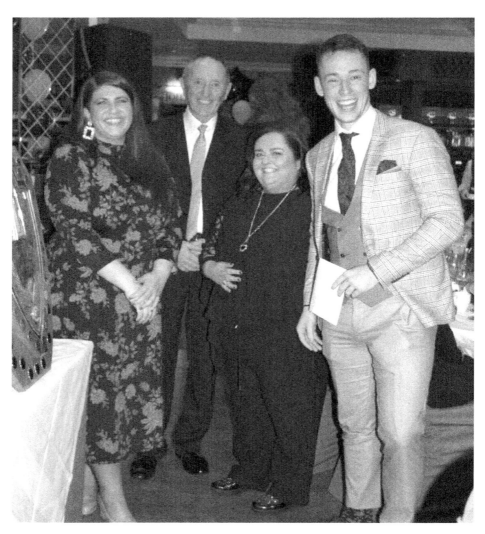

Jack Morgan, on right, best dressed man at the Rock & Rose Victory Social at the Rose Hotel Tralee on 22nd February 2020 is pictured with Mary McQuinn, Billy Ryle and Siobhán Power

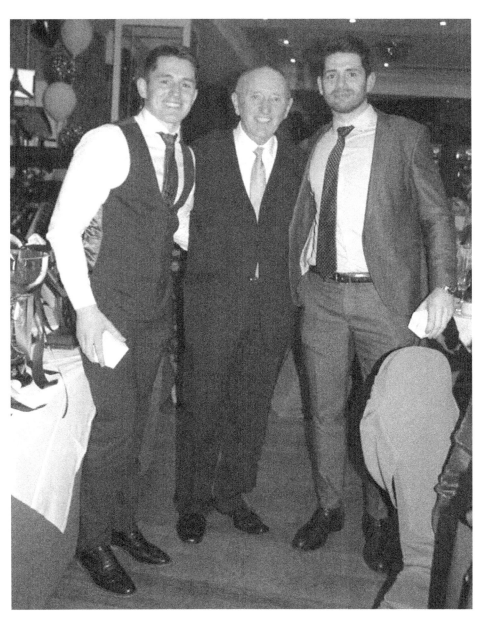

Ronan, left, and Barry Shanahan receive their medals from Billy Ryle at the Rock & Rose Victory Social at the Rose Hotel Tralee on 22nd February 2020

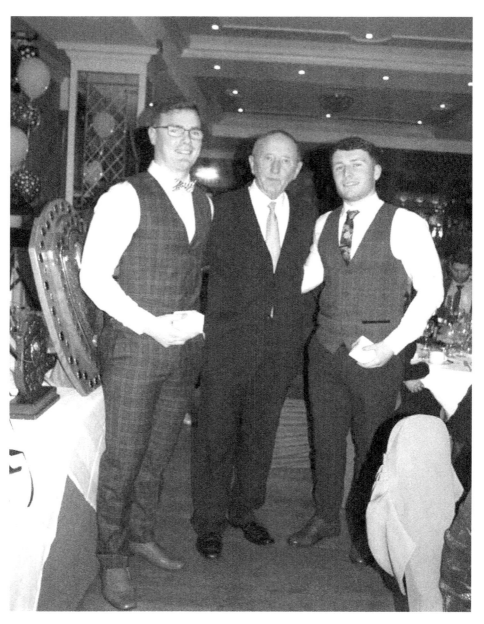

Greg Horan, left, and Conor Jordan receive their medals from Billy Ryle at the Rock & Rose Victory Social at the Rose Hotel Tralee on 22nd February 2020

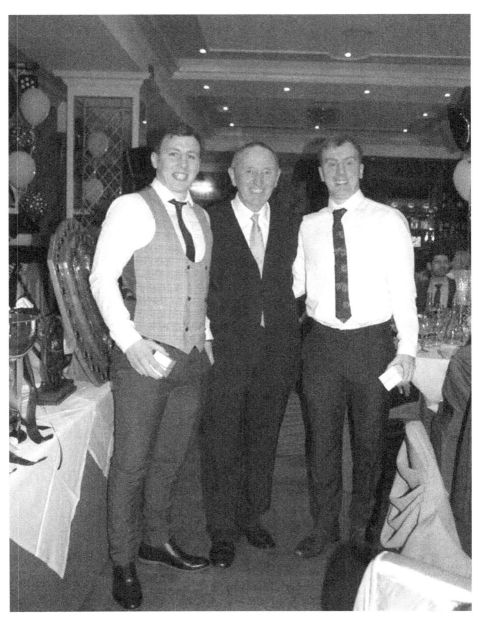

Darragh O'Brien, left and Shane O'Callaghan receive their medals from Billy Ryle at the Rock & Rose Victory Social at the Rose Hotel Tralee on 22nd February 2020

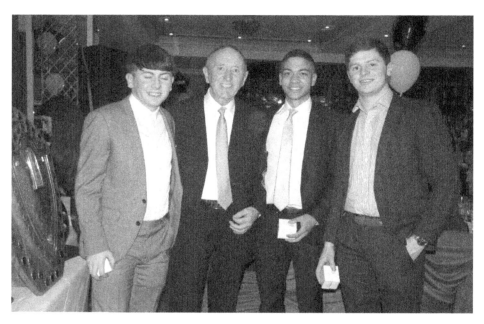

Shane Kelliher, left, Brandon Patterson and Shane Walsh receive their medals from Billy Ryle at the Rock & Rose Victory at the Rose Hotel Tralee on 22nd February 2020

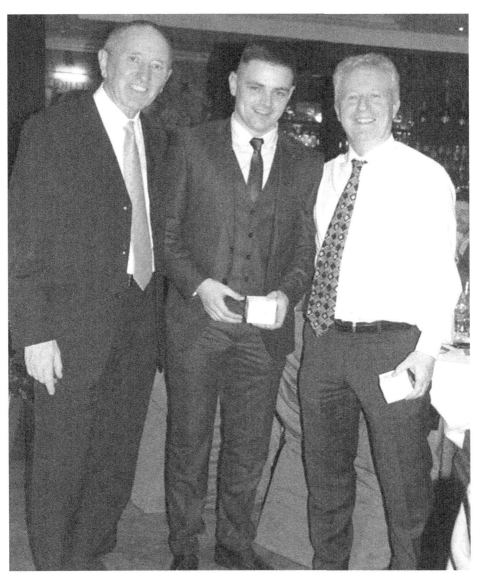

Colin Griffin, centre and Éamonn O'Reilly, right, on behalf of his son Ciarán, receive their medals from Billy Ryle at the Rock & Rose Victory Social at the Rose Hotel Tralee on 22nd February 2020

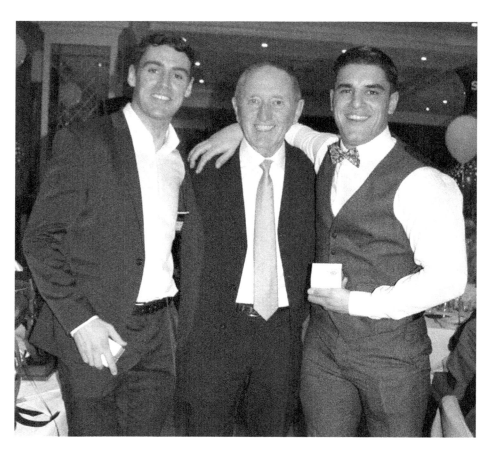

Fiachna Mangan, left and Wayne Guthrie, right, receive their medals from Billy Ryle at the Rock & Rose Victory Social at the Rose Hotel Tralee on 22nd February 2020

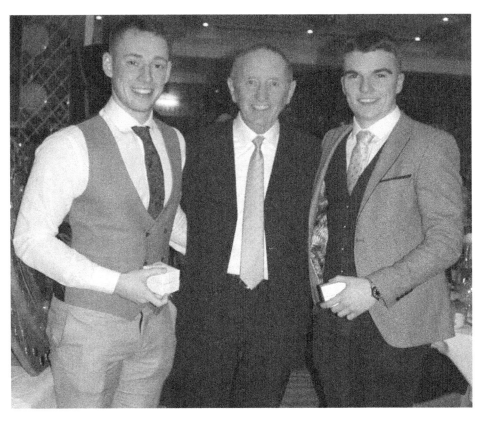

Jack Morgan, left and Dylan Casey, right, receive their medals from Billy Ryle at the Rock & Rose Victory Social at the Rose Hotel Tralee on 22nd February 2020

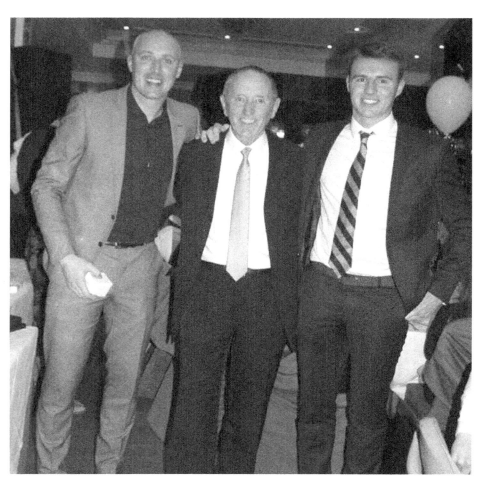

Kieran Donaghy, left and Michael O'Donnell, right, receive their medals from Billy Ryle at the Rock & Rose Victory Social at the Rose Hotel Tralee on 22nd February 2020

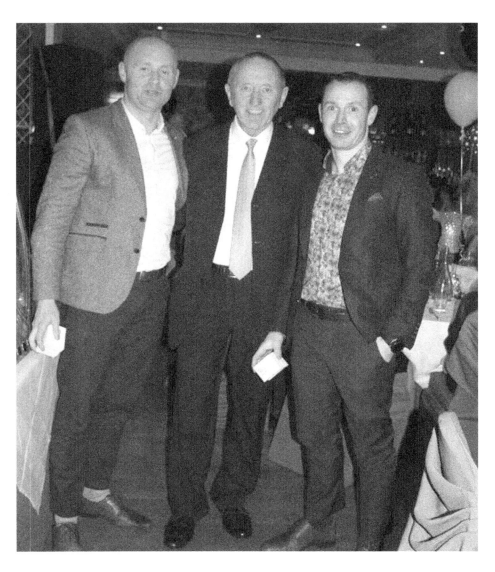

Darragh Long, left and Mikey Collins, right, receive their medals from Billy Ryle at the Rock & Rose Victory Social at the Rose Hotel Tralee on 22nd February 2020

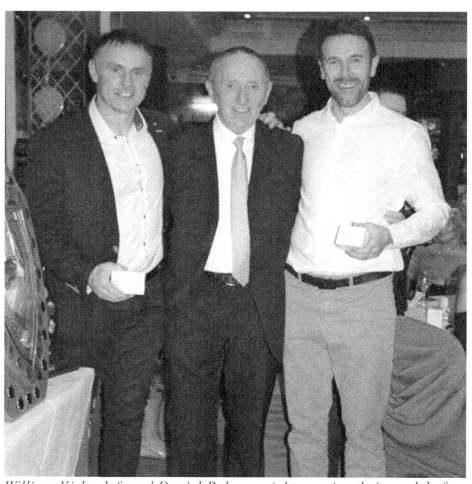

William Kirby, left and Daniel Bohane, right, receive their medals from Billy Ryle at the Rock & Rose Victory Social at the Rose Hotel Tralee on 22nd February 2020

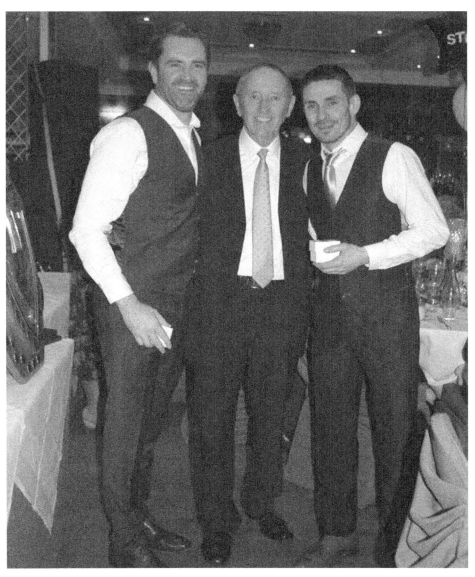

Ger Teahan, left and Tommy Costello, right, receive their medals from Billy Ryle at the Rock & Rose Victory Social at the Rose Hotel Tralee on 22nd February 2020

CHAPTER FIFTEEN

LOCKDOWN

My next appointment in Cork with Mister Flynn was scheduled for the 29th May 2020 when the country was in lockdown. My eye sight was reasonably good and the cataract surgery had improved the vision in my right eye. I was expecting my surgeries to proceed during 2020 but the pressure put on the public health service more or less put paid to that.

During the 2km restriction I was unable to pursue my favourite hobby of sea swimming. Even though I have a lovely sea view from my back garden, the bathing slip in Fenit where I regularly swim is about 4km from my house. I had decided to comply fully with the public health guidelines as it was the right thing to do. My wife, Sheila, our dog Jake and I did a daily walk along a circular route which kept us within our 2km distance from home. While I am not a natural walker, I really took to the routine and looked forward to it each day, hail, rain or shine. All the neighbours were doing likewise so we were all criss-crossing each other as some of us took a clock-wise direction and others went in the opposite direction. Sheila, Jake and myself varied our direction as the mood took us.

I longed for the day when it would be safe to lift the various restrictions and return to normal living. I often wondered if the normality we were used to would ever be restored or were we facing into a totally different type of lifestyle and living. Whatever, I made a promise to myself that if I came safely through the coronavirus pandemic, I would never again take my love of exercise and sport for granted. Being housebound and confined to short walks within the 2km radius, I missed the invigorating walks with my wife along the lonely Banna Strand, where Roger Casement came ashore on Good Friday, 1916. I missed my daily swim in the clear blue sea of the Wild Atlantic Way at Fenit bathing slip. I missed supporting my beloved Austin Stacks GAA Club in their football matches and I missed the live sports reports in the media.

I was very pleased when the restriction was stretched to 5km from home as it allowed me to resume swimming in the sea at Fenit. The daily swim was wonderful and my fitness in the water improved with each passing day. I regretted that many of my swimming colleagues were unable to join me in Fenit as they lived more than 5km from Fenit Village. My passion for reading sustained me during the lockdown and I enjoyed spending time in our garden, cutting grass, trimming hedges and all the minor chores that go with gardening.

My professional life came to a halt. I made a decision, despite many requests, not to provide virtual career and educational consultations. I have always been protective of the confidential nature of my work. I'm a face-to-face communicator who considers body language important in building rapport with a client. Besides, I had no control over anybody who might be silently listening in to a consultation off-screen.

One particular event which I thoroughly enjoyed was the Austin Stacks Run4Pieta, which was organised by our Club's dynamic Vice-Chairman, Eamonn O Reilly and his dedicated team. They did a brilliant job of organising the Austin Stacks Run4Pieta over one weekend, from 7.30pm on Friday, 8th May to 7.30pm on Saturday, 9th May, 2020. Club members ran, jogged and walked a 4km journey for a deserving cause while adhering to public health guidelines. From the moment the fundraiser was launched on our club's website our members, supporters and friends began very generously donating to the Pieta charity. People continued to donate on our website for some weeks and dug deep for this worthy fundraiser. Every cent collected went directly to Pieta to help finance their invaluable work. Pieta House provides free counselling for people suffering from suicidal ideation, engaging in self-harm and those who have been bereaved by suicide. It was wonderful that the event provided some much-welcomed club activity. Even though it was a virtual event and we all did the walk in our own time while complying with the restrictions, it helped to bond the club members, supporters and friends

The Club Executive Committee continued to keep in touch via video link with all matters off the field. We hoped to have everything ready to go as soon as the health experts gave us the all clear to resume activities. The club was in the safe hands of our various administrative committees even though all was quiet in Connolly Park. So, in an online message to our members, I encouraged them to get out and enjoy exercise in accordance with the health guidelines, to practise the skills in the back garden and to keep in touch with each other in order to keep morale high. I was hopeful that there would still be a lot of football played in 2020 despite the lockdown.

On our car journey to Cork on the 29th May 2020, Sheila and I were stopped at a Garda checkpoint. We were asked for the purpose of our journey and we were able to produce evidence of my 12.15pm appointment with Mr Flynn. We fully appreciated the need for checkpoint as a means of preventing people from unrestricted travel in dangerous times.

It had been five months since I had cataract surgery in my right eye. Mister Flynn said my vision was at a level where he would find it difficult to make a strong recommendation to have a corneal graft. He suggested that I update my glasses and use hypertonic saline drops. He expected that there would be some deterioration of the Fuchs Dystrophy over time, which would make the decision on corneal graft easier. I was given a further appointment for the 27th November 2020. I now realised that the plan was to concentrate on my right eye rather than to proceed with cataract surgery in my left eye. That seemed to me to be a sensible plan as it would hopefully provide me with reasonably good sight in one eye. I assumed then that cataract surgery and a corneal transplant would be done on my left eye sometime after the corneal transplant in my right eye.

As my vision wasn't being over stretched due to suspension of football matches and the restrictions on driving, I wasn't complaining. I was quite happy to follow Mr Flynn's timeline for me. Of course, all those involved in healthcare were waging a huge battle against the Covid-19 and there were many people who needed their expertise ahead of myself. Somewhere deep down inside me, I was happy to keep away from hospital while the pandemic was causing havoc.

Dr O'Regan prescribed reading glasses for me and I began, primarily, to read books with enlarged print. I made the most of my situation realising that many people were far worse off than myself. Lives were being lost to the virus. Families were suffering bereavement and were being traumatised by the isolated and lonely deaths of their loved ones. I was fully set on making the most of summer 2020 until my next visit to the Elysian on 27th November 2020 almost a year after cataract surgery on my right eye.

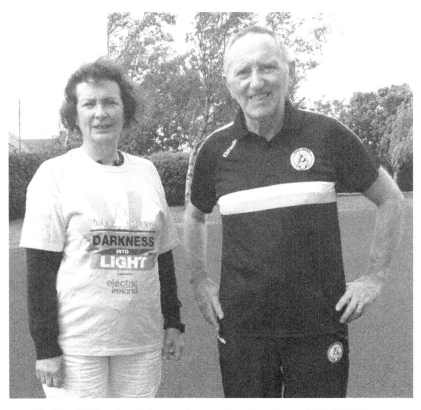

Billy & Sheila Ryle took part in the virtual Walk4Pieta on the 9th May 2020

CHAPTER SIXTEEN

A COVID FUNERAL

On the 8th May 2020, the Austin Stack Club lost one of its most loyal members. Des Hurley passed away quietly and because of the Covid-19 restrictions, his funeral took place before we learned of his passing. So, on the 15th May 2020, I invited some of my senior colleagues, Mairéad Fernane, Eddie Barrett, Martin Collins and Tadgh McMahon to join me for a short ceremony at the grave in Rath Cemetery, Tralee. I also felt it appropriate to invite Simon Foley and Tom Baker, two close friends of Des along with Des' and my own personal friend, Paddy Kissane. Des, Paddy and myself are lifelong swimming buddies at the bathing slip in Fenit.

I placed a bouquet of flowers on the grave on behalf of Austin Stacks and I delivered the graveside oration, published below. We collectively sang that great Irish rallying song, 'Oró sé do bheatha abhaile'. Mairéad then beautifully read our club poem, 'The boys from the top of the Rock.' We chatted around the grave, observing social distance, where we informally exchanged happy memories of Des. It was our tribute to a great Rock man, in a less than normal time which was imposed on us by the Covid -19 virus.

"It's often said that when the Angel of death calls, he returns to Heaven with three connected souls. Austin Stacks can vouch for that statement as in recent months we have lost three valued members, Seán Murphy, Timmy Sheehan and now Des Hurley. Des passed away quietly on Friday, 8th May 2020 and had a private burial on Saturday, 9th May. He went to his grave without fuss or fanfare, which epitomised the calm way in which he lived his life. Des' passing left unfinished business for the Austin Stacks Club. We had no time to mourn his passing. We got no opportunity to say goodbye. We were unable to be with him on his final journey. So, we gather today at his graveside to bid a proper farewell to our friend, neighbour and colleague, a committed Rockie for seventy-two years.

Born in 1935, Des grew up in Pembroke Street in a family steeped in Rock tradition. He wore a minor jersey for the first time in 1951, aged just sixteen years of age, at a time when The Rock was ravaged by emigration. During the next few years, Des often had to play minor, junior and senior football in the same year such was the shortage of players in the club. Austin Stacks was in the doldrums during the 40's and 50's. It took a small dedicated group of people to keep the club alive during a challenging economic period. Des felt very proud that, in the worst of times, Austin Stacks never failed to field a team or fulfil a fixture.

Des' promising football career was cut short in 1955 when he was forced to emigrate to London in pursuit of employment. He worked hard and learned a great deal about the construction industry before the call of home drew him back to Tralee in the early seventies. He opened the Rose Restaurant in Russell St, where he ran a very successful business. Indeed, many a club meeting was held over tea and scones in the Restaurant. Des was an astute business man, particularly in the construction and property industries where he established a reputation as a man who could be trusted to deliver what he promised. Des was totally committed to rebuilding the reputation of Tralee as a progressive business town and, of course, to the development of our new pitch and facilities at Connolly Park.

On his return from London, Des immediately immersed himself in the Rock Club. His playing days were over but he was elected to the executive committee of the club where his personal drive and business acumen were invaluable in the revival of Austin Stacks, both on and off the field. Des was overjoyed in 1973 when Austin Stacks won the Kerry Senior Football Championship after thirty-seven barren years. He loved the Rock Club throughout his life. He was a loyal supporter of Austin Stacks and Kerry right to the end. He got great satisfaction from our successes down through the years. 'The Stacks are back and we're here to stay,' was his mantra. Des was especially excited by our current talented squad which won both the County Senior Club Football Championship and the County Senior Football League Division One last year under the stewardship of Wayne Quillinan, our senior team Manager. He was confident that the Holy Grail, the County Senior Football Championship was a realistic target for the club this year. He didn't live long enough to find out but we'll do everything we can to win that title for him if play ever resumes this year.

Des had another great passion – Fenit. He was a life-long swimmer and he loved his regular dip at the bathing slip. Des, Paddy Kissane, who is with us today and myself spent many wonderful afternoons basking in the sun and discussing the major current affairs of the day. Invariably, the discussion always reverted back to Rock and Kerry football. Des lived a simple and modest life. He made the most of every day before being laid low by his final illness. He was his own man and loved living in Mounthawk, mid-way between his two great sporting loves in Fenit and Connolly Park. He never fully retired from his business interests but he did eventually treat himself to a campervan, which gave him the freedom to head off to Clare, West Cork or Galway or wherever, when the humour took him. He was always back in Tralee whenever the Rock or Kerry were due to play. In fact, in recent years, the campervan seemed to be parked in Fenit for the entire summer so that Des could enjoy the good weather and sell the beauty of Kerry and Fenit, in particular, to all who crossed his path. Des' ideal tourist was one who spent big, loved football and was prepared to listen to him wax lyrical about John O Keeffe, Ger Power, Paddy Moriarty, Kieran Donaghy and one of his favourites, Tommy Bracker O Regan.

We had no chance to say goodbye. The coronavirus pandemic denied us of that opportunity. Matches were postponed for the past few months. Fenit carpark was locked down. There was no getting together in town for a cup of coffee and a chat. We were told to stay at home. We did as we were told. We didn't realise how ill Des was. He didn't tell us. He was private and dignified to the end.

But Des is not alone today. His friends and colleagues are at his graveside to pay tribute to a life well lived, to thank him for his selfless dedication to his beloved Rock Club. We are here today on behalf of many more, who are not allowed join us due to health and safety regulations, to bid farewell to a genuine 'auld stock of the Rock.' We return his immortal soul to his God. Des will always be fondly remembered, but the time has come to let him go. It's time to say goodbye. So farewell, old friend. May you rest in peace and may the green sod rest lightly on your gentle soul."

I was at hand on Monday night 8th June 2020 to relaunch the Austin Stacks Hurling and Football Club Lotto in a concerted effort to replenish our funds, which were depleted by the pandemic. I also availed of the opportunity in my speech, published below, to acknowledge the disciplined response of our entire club membership to the Croke Park Directives and Government National Public Health Guidelines in the fight against the Coronavirus pandemic. I also wholeheartedly welcome the news that GAA activity was to resume in the next few weeks. But the evening was all about launching the online lotto and paying tribute to our dedicated Club Lotto Committee.

"I'd like to welcome everybody to our Club Grounds, Connolly Park, Tralee, for the online launch of our club fundraising Lotto," I began. "Before getting to the Lotto, I want to acknowledge the disciplined response of our entire club membership to the Croke Park Directives and Government National Public Health Guidelines in the fight against the coronavirus pandemic. The past three months have been very difficult, especially for our players, from the youngest to the oldest, who were denied the joy of training and the thrill of competition. But we are nearly there and Austin Stacks will continue to comply fully with Croke Park Directives and Public Health Guidelines every step of the way. I wholeheartedly welcome the news that GAA activity is to resume in the next few weeks. According to the 'Safe Return to Gaelic Games Roadmap' issued by the GAA on Friday, 5th June 2020, all of our pitches will reopen on the 29th June, but all indoor facilities except sanitized toilet facilities must remain closed. Non-contact training will begin for our players in small groups. All forms of team and group training will begin on the 20th July. Indoor facilities must still remain closed. Club competitions for all grades will begin on the 31st July.

I want the word to go out loud and clear from Connolly Park – Austin Stacks is raring to go and can hardly wait to get started. We are ready, willing and able. It's time to let the games begin. We saw the best of our club during the lockdown beginning with our Club Community Response. This wonderful initiative by our gallant band of volunteers meant that no one in need was left unaided, alone or isolated. Our young team members willingly took on the tasks that housebound people couldn't do for themselves. By their many good deeds and fundraising initiatives, our members proved that Austin Stacks is more than a club. It's also a caring community. I'd like to mention just a few of those fundraisers. Club Vice-Chairman, Eamonn O Reilly and his dedicated team organised the Austin Stacks Run4Pieta on Friday/Saturday, 8th/9th May. Club members ran or walked a 4km journey for a deserving cause while adhering to public health guidelines. Gally's Gallop, a 200km run, was a fundraiser organised by senior footballer, Eoghan Galvin for Kerry Cancer Support. Club Executive Committee member, Mairéad Fernane undertook a head-shave fundraiser for Kerry Hospice Foundation. Collectively, those three events alone have raised in excess of €20,000 to date, with donations still coming in.

I want to thank the Club's Executive Committee for keeping the club ticking over by way of our virtual meetings via Zoom. I'd like to mention Club Secretary Elma Nix, in particular, who diligently kept us up-to-date with all developments and events. I want to thank our Senior Team Manager Wayne Quillinan, Ladies Club Chairperson Bernie Mannix, Juvenile Club Chairman Tim McMahon, Coaching & Games Development Officer Éamonn O'Reilly and all of our team mentors who kept in regular touch with our players with fitness and drill instructions. This initiative kept morale and enthusiasm sky high amongst the players during the lockdown. They are all looking forward to resuming training and games.

Field Committee Chairman, Jim Naughton and his willing volunteers have done an outstanding job of grounds maintenance and painting, even enlisting our fellow club member, Mike O Donnell to adorn the area with his beautiful mural art. I'd like to say a special thank you to our Clubman of the Year, Noel O Connell for his invaluable advice and assistance during the lockdown. My thanks to Finance Committee Chairman, Nial Shanahan, Club Treasurer Mike Tangney and Club Assistant Treasurer Anne Marie Healy and the Finance Committee for managing to stretch our limited finances during the past three months. I'd also like to acknowledge the generosity, in very difficult times, of our main club Sponsor, Kirby's Brogue Inn Bar and Restaurant and our Ladies' Club sponsor Terry's Butchers. They stood shoulder to shoulder with us in the dark days of COVID -19. We will, hopefully, repay them with silverware in the good days to come.

But this evening is all about our dedicated Club Lotto Committee – Nial Shanahan, Bernie Mannix, Carmel O Neill, Brendan O Regan, Martin Collins and John Breen who were first out of the starting blocks by getting the offline Lotto up and running last Monday night. The three months loss of Lotto income was a big setback, so well done to the Lotto Committee for reactivating this vital fundraiser so speedily. If we have learned anything during the lockdown, it is that we have to adapt to modern methods of communication or we'll be left behind. Tonight. we are taking a major step in that direction by making our Lotto available online. This is an exciting initiative by our Lotto Committee to reach out to a much wider playing audience locally, nationally and worldwide. Playing the Austin Stacks Club Fundraising Lotto online will be very straight forward. It takes just six easy steps to play. All you need do is visit our club Website, Facebook Page or Twitter Account, click on the lotto links and follow the steps.

The current JACKPOT is €13,400. There are five consolation prizes of €20 in each weekly draw. The weekly draw takes place each Monday evening. Online tickets purchased up to 6pm on a Monday will be included in that evening's Lotto draw. Tickets purchased online after 6pm on a Monday will be included in the following Monday's Lotto draw. Results of the Austin Stacks GAA Club fundraising Lotto draw are published weekly on our website, club notes and social media platforms. So, in anticipation of a great boost for our depleted club finances, it's a great pleasure for me as Chairman of Austin Stacks

Hurling and Football Club to declare our online fundraising Lotto to be officially launched. The Best of luck to all Lotto players!"

I'm delighted to say that the Lotto has gone from strength during the past few years and continues to be a regular source of income for Austin Stacks. As well as a substantial Jackpot, there are five consolation prizes of €20 in each weekly draw. The weekly draw continues to take place each Monday evening.

There was great joy when the GAA circulated its safe return to play guidelines on the 5th June 2020. Having been locked down for the previous three months, everybody looked forward to the return of GAA games. The players were chomping at the bit to resume training, club officials were anxious to get moving on the administrative side and the supporters were looking forward to a comprehensive fixture schedule. The return was carefully phased in with strict guidelines applying to each phase. Austin Stacks meticulously enforced the guidelines attached with each phase and the club was opened up for the resumption of play. Training gradually progressed from no physical contact to full contact. All forms of team and group training began on the 20th July. Indoor facilities still remained closed. Club competitions for all grades began on the 31st July. The Senior Club Championship was to be made up of two groups of four teams each and the winners of each group would meet in the final. There would be an open draw of sixteen teams in the Kerry Senior Football Championship which would be run on a straight knock out basis. There would be no second chance and there would be no room for a slip up in the Senior Championship of 2020. Because the divisional sides would have less time to train and bond due to the late reopening of the season, I had high hopes of Austin Stacks winning the County Senior Championship in 2020. But for now, it was time to focus on the Senior Club Championship.

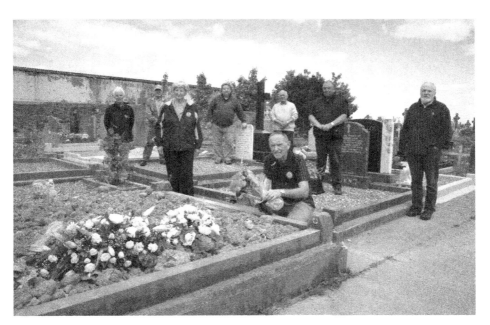

A Covid Farewell: Billy Ryle, on behalf of Austin Stacks GAA Club, Tralee places a bouquet of flowers on the grave of Des Hurley in Rath Cemetery, Tralee on the 15th May 2020, Standing, from left, Tadgh Mc Mahon, Martin Collins, Mairéad Fernane, Eddie Barrett, Simon Foley, Tom Baker and Paddy Kissane

CHAPTER SEVENTEEN

THE BRACKER 100KM WALK

Early in my Chairmanship, I became aware of a major access issue in our facilities. Supporters, who were wheelchair bound or unsteady under foot were unable to access the far side of our main pitch where Rock supports usually congregate. Our main pitch is perpendicular to our second pitch, known as the Nun's Field and supporters use the grass margin between the two pitches to cross to the far side of the main pitch. The rough surface was unsuitable for wheelchair access and uneven under foot for the elderly and those unsteady in their stance. The footfall also tended to damage the playing surfaces and many people tended to drift on to the playing pitches as they came and went. When the surface was soft after wet weather the pitches suffered damage and needed repair. So, in order to resolve both issues, I decided to do a personal fundraising walk to have a new concrete path laid between the pitches.

The walk would be 100km over a ten-day period on the Bracker O'Regan Road, named in honour of Martin Bracker O'Regan, who was one of the club's and Kerry's best and most colourful players. Martin coined the immortal phrase, 'put me on the forty-five yards line and build the team around me!' There is a beautiful monument located on the road in memory of Martin. I enlisted the help of a few friends and set up an online Go-Fund-Me account. The Bracker 100km fundraising walk was launched at the Bracker Monument on Monday, 13th July 2020 by Austin Stacks and Kerry football legend, Mikey Sheehy. My own words of welcome and thanks follow below. Members of Martin Bracker O'Regan's family were guests at the launch. Fr. Padraig Walsh PP, Church of Our Lady and Saint Brendan, Upper Rock St, Tralee blessed the Bracker Monument, myself the walker, and also imparted a general blessing to all present. I was pleasantly surprise by the amount of money that was contributed at the launch.

"It's my great pleasure" I said "to welcome everybody to the launch of The Bracker 100km fundraising walk here at the Martin Bracker O'Regan Memorial Monument. A very special welcome to our own superstar, Mikey Sheehy who is honouring us by launching the fundraiser. I'd like to welcome Fr. Pádraig Walsh PP, Church of Our Lady and St. Brendan, who will bless the Bracker Monument and impart a blessing to all gathered here. I welcome the members of Martin Bracker O'Regan's family who are with us this evening.

The walk is dedicated to the memory of Martin Bracker O Regan, one of Austin Stacks and Kerry's finest footballers. I'd like to avail of the opportunity to thank those who assisted me in organising this fundraiser and tonight's launch, especially Noel O'Connell, Martin O'Regan, Éamonn O'Reilly, Denis O'Regan and Mairéad Fernane. The purpose of the walk is to raise badly needed funds to lay a new path behind the main pitch to prevent footfall damage on the pitches and to facilitate disability access to the far terrace in Connolly Park. So, I'm appealing to all club members and supporters at home in Ireland and around the world to donate to the online fundraiser.

Every donation, big and small, will be appreciated. Also, please share the link, https://www.gofundme.com/f/the-bracker-100km, as widely as possible to help us reach our target. I'll walk 100km on Bracker O Regan Road over a ten-day period between next Friday and Sunday week – two sessions per day on the path, beginning and ending at the Bracker Monument - a 6km walk beginning at 10am and a 4km walk beginning at 3pm. Please join me at any stage for a lap or two as I never like to walk alone!

In a beautiful profile of Mikey Sheehy in our Club's Centenary Book, our Club PRO, Martin Collins wrote, and I quote, 'Mikey Sheehy was arguably the Club's and possibly Kerry's greatest footballer winning five County Championship medals, seven County League titles, a

Munster and All Ireland Club Title in 1976/77. Along with Club mate Ger Power, Mikey won a record eight All Ireland Senior Medals.'

In your own time, read Martin's outstanding profile of Mikey to fully appreciate what a talented footballer we have in our midst. Mikey Sheehy and Martin Bracker O'Regan were friends and neighbours. They had great respect for each other – each person maintaining that the other was the better footballer. But as we all know they were both superstars of The Rock and Kerry. When I asked the O'Regan family who they would like to launch the Bracker 100km fundraising walk there was only one answer - Mikey. So, it's my great pleasure to invite Mikey to cut the ribbon to formally launch the Bracker 100km fundraising walk. When Mikey has cut the ribbon, it will be my pleasure to hand over to a man who is walking on air for the last few weeks with a broad smile on his face since his beloved Liverpool won the English Premier League title – Fr. Pádraig Walsh."

Mikey was fulsome in his praise for Martin and the O'Regan family and he said that he was delighted to launch the walk. He wished me well on the road and appealed to one and all to support the fundraising effort. Mikey said that our pitches in Connolly Park should be disability access friendly so that all supporters could enjoy the games. He admitted that he was a great fan of the late Martin Bracker and he conceded that Martin was a much better footballer than himself. While we all admired Mickey's customary modesty, we felt that the two superstars stood side by side in the pantheon of Austin Stack and Kerry football greats. Fr, Pádraig then blessed the Martin Bracker O'Regan Memorial Monument and all of us present. He wished me will on the walk and promised to keep me in his prayers.

It was a fabulous launch on a perfect evening. I was so grateful to Mikey and Fr. Pádraig for doing the honours at the event. The large attendance at the launch gave me a great boost and filled me with the self-belief that I could accomplish the task I had set for myself. Now that the ribbon was cut and the money was flowing in, there was no turning back! I began walking on Friday 17th July 2020 and completed the walk on Sunday 26th July. I walked two sessions per day on the path, beginning and ending at the Bracker Monument, a 6km walk beginning at 10am and a 4km walk beginning at 3pm. I kept reminding one and all through conventional and social media that The Bracker 100km was a worldwide online fundraiser to pay for a path behind the main pitch. The new path would prevent footfall damage on the pitches and would facilitate disability access to the far terrace in Connolly Park.

By Tuesday evening, I was halfway in The Bracker100km fundraising walk. Weather conditions were excellent and my road was being shortened by the people who turned up to walk with me. The waves and horn blasts as people walked, cycled or drove past added to the banter on the walk. I encouraged more people to join me on the walk during the remaining days. I reminded them that I'd be at the Bracker Monument every day until the following Sunday at 10am and 3pm.

It was all about the money to build a path with disability access, so I kept on appealing to people to donate. Over the final few days, I tried hard to convert promises of donation into hard cash. I asked people to make the donation immediately lest they forget. Every single donation, big or small, would be gratefully accepted and would help to make life a bit easier for those who want to enjoy the games in comfort.

Day eight, Friday, was our wettest day yet. Conditions were good in early morning but the heavy rain fell as we walked. Thankfully, the rain had passed before session two in the afternoon. There were just two days to go on our 100km journey. We had planned a ceremonial finish at The Bracker Memorial Monument on Sunday afternoon to mark the completion of 100km. The event would conclude with a few stories, poems and songs associated with Martin Bracker O'Regan.

I completed The Bracker 100km fundraising walk on Sunday afternoon, 26th July 2020. I did the regular 6km session on Sunday morning and the twentieth session, the final 4km session in the afternoon. It was a great feeling to step over the line for the last time. I was exhausted after ten consecutive days of walking and looking forward to returning to my favourite leisure activity, sea swimming in Fenit. I was blessed with good weather, with only one shower in all twenty sessions. Otherwise, it was sunshine all the way.

I mightn't have made it to the end of the 100km journey without the support of my faithful band of walkers who sustained me with stories, laughter and companionship over the ten days. Among them were Mairéad Fernane, Tim Guiheen, Noel O'Connell, Tim Slattery, Liz and Denis O' Regan, Martin Collins, Kevin Barry, Tim Lynch, John Tobin, Tadgh and Ann McMahon, Carmel and Martin O' Regan. I owed them a very sincere debt of gratitude. They even allowed me to be first to cross the finishing line, which was a lovely gesture. Our group shared a lovely celebration of poetry, stories and good humour at The Bracker Memorial Monument at the end of the 100km walk to bring down the curtain on a memorable ten-day event. It was very special and I will always fondly remember the experience.

The Organising Committee of the 'Bracker 100km fundraising walk' presented the proceeds raised from the walk to the Austin Stacks GAA Club on Saturday, 19th September 2020 at the Bracker Memorial Monument on Bracker O'Regan Road. I was chuffed and surprised when the O'Regan family presented me with a framed copy of the famous poem, 'On Bracker's Road,' which was composed by Jimmy O'Regan, as a memento of the occasion. I will always treasure it as a fond reminder of a wonderful ten days on the Bracker O'Regan Road.

I also availed of the opportunity to once again thank everybody who contributed to the recent fundraising walk. In particular I thanked the organising committee of Noel O'Connell, Martin O'Regan, Mairéad Fernane, Éamonn O'Reilly and Denis O'Regan for their generous help and support before and during the walk. I expressed my gratitude to the people who walked some laps with me during the twenty sessions over ten days. The moral support, banter and laughter in their company made the journey very enjoyable and less demanding. I thanked Mikey Sheehy who launched the event and those who provided the story-telling and poetry at the conclusion of a memorable event. The fundraiser grossed a sum of €3570. After the deduction of a fee of €117.80, the organising committee was delighted to present Nial

Shanahan, Chairman of the Club Finance Committee with a cheque for €3452.20. This money went towards the provision of a path to improve access in Connolly Park for people who are disabled or unsteady in movement. The story of laying and opening the path will be told in Chapters 25 and 30.

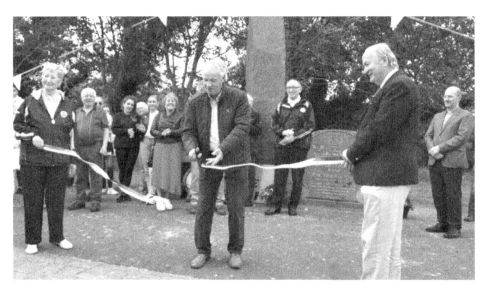

Mikey Sheehy cuts the ribbon to launch The Bracker 100km Fundraising Walk on the 13th July 2020. Mairéad Fernane and Jim Finucane hold the tape. Watching on, from left, are Jimmy O'Regan, Carmel O'Regan, Billy Ryle and Fr Pádraig Walsh

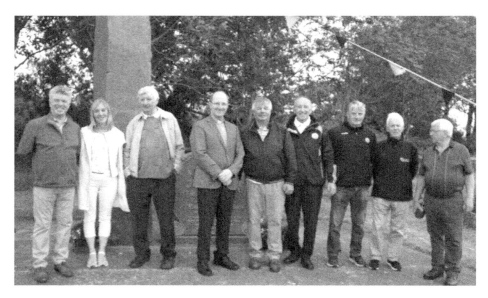

At the launch of The Bracker 100km Fundraising Walk at the Martin Bracker O'Regan Monument on the 13th July 2020 were from left, Denis, Mary and Tommy O'Regan, Fr Pádraig Walsh, Martin O'Regan, Billy Ryle, Noel O'Connell, Tadgh McMahon and Jimmy O'Regan

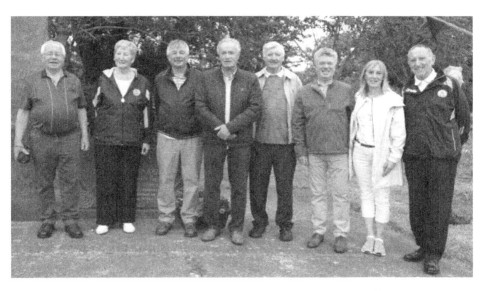

At the launch of The Bracker 100km Fundraising Walk at the Martin Bracker O'Regan Monument on the 13th July 2020 were from left, Jimmy O'Regan, Mairéad Fernane, Martin O'Regan, Mikey Sheehy, Tommy, Denis, Mary O'Regan and Billy Ryle

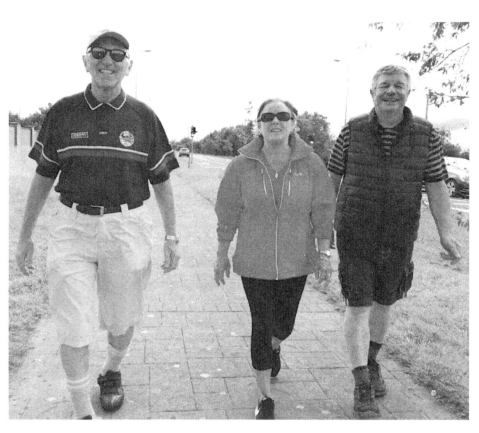

Billy Ryle, left, on The Bracker 100km Fundraising Walk with Carmel and Martin O'Regan on the 23rd July 2020

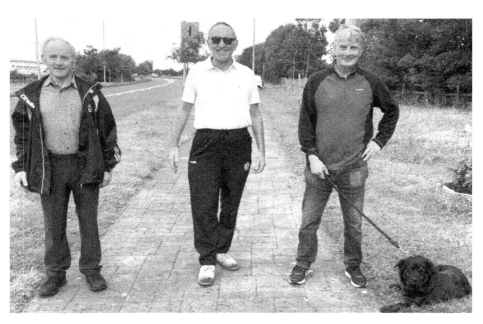

Billy Ryle, centre, on The Bracker 100km Fundraising Walk with Tim Slattery, left, and Noel O'Connell on the 18th July 2020

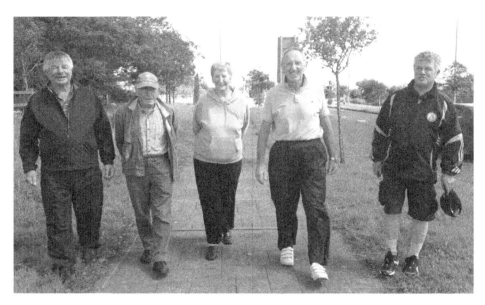

On the The Bracker 100km Fundraising Walk on the 25th July 2020 were, from left, Martin O'Regan, Martin Collins, Mairéad Fernane, Billy Ryle and Denis O'Regan

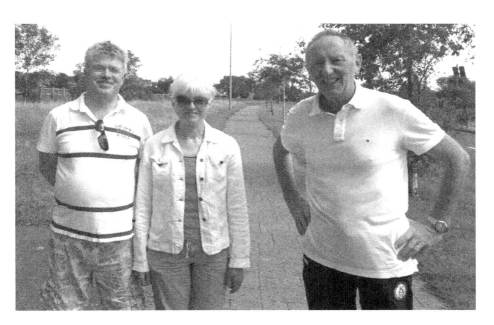

Billy Ryle, right, on The Bracker 100km Fundraising Walk with Liz and Denis O'Regan on the 18th July 2020

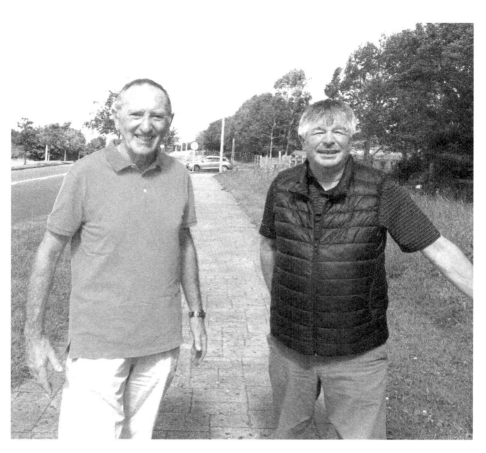

Billy Ryle, left, and Martin O'Regan on The Bracker 100km Fundraising Walk on the 19th July 2020

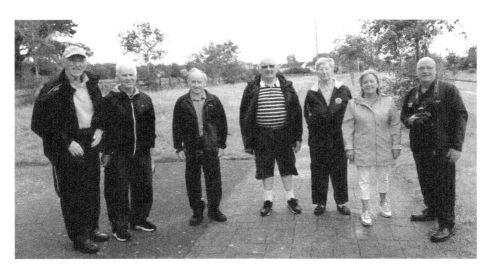

Paddy Whyte, Photographer with Kerry's Eye Newspaper, on right, who was present to record the final day of The Bracker 100km Fundraising Walk on the 25th July 2020, is pictured with, from left, Billy Ryle, Tadgh Mc Mahon, Tim Slattery, Tim Guiheen, Mairéad Fernane and Carmel O'Regan

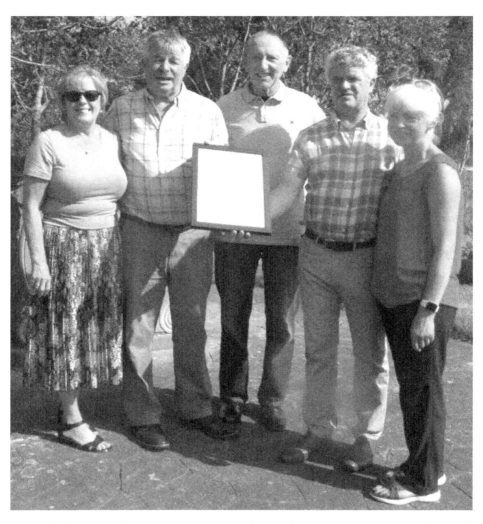

From left, Carmel, Martin, Denis and Liz O'Regan presented Billy Ryle, centre, with a framed copy of the famous poem, On Bracker's Road, on the 19th September 2020

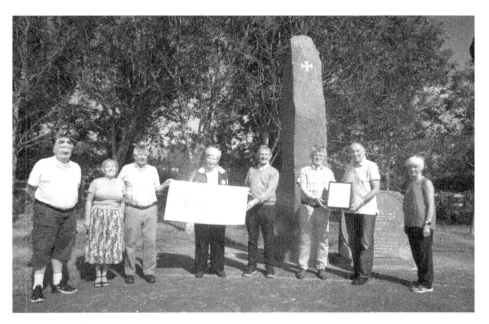

On the 19th September 2020 Martin O'Regan and Mairéad Fernane, on behalf of the Organising Committee, presented the proceeds of The The Bracker 100km Fundraising Walk to Nial Shanahan, Chairman of Austin Stacks Finance Committee and Denis O'Regan presented Billy Ryle with a memento of the walk. Pictured, from left: Tim Guiheen, Carmel and Martin O'Regan, Mairéad Fernane, Nial Shanahan, Denis O'Regan, Billy Ryle and Liz O'Regan

CHAPTER EIGHTEEN

CLUB TITLE BUT CHAMPIONSHIP EXIT

After months of inactivity, Austin Stacks Senior football team began the defence of the Senior Club Championship title, which it had won in 2019, long before the Covid- 19 virus was ever heard of. We travelled to Annascaul on Saturday evening, 25th July 2020 with high hopes of getting off to a good start in this competition against Dingle. After a very competitive game the sides finished level on a score of 1-12 each. As it subsequently turned out, the point we earned in Annascaul would prove to be priceless on our road to the final.

The Annascaul Club had everything organized to perfection on the night. Hosting the fixture in those very challenging times for contact sport wasn't an easy ask. With only two hundred spectators allowed to attend the game, many of our loyal supporters were unable to be accommodated. I was very hopeful that the attendance would be increased to five hundred in the not-to-distant future. I was delighted with the good result in our first game of this competition. I was confident that we could achieve an even better result in our second-round game against Kilcummin. That fixture was scheduled for our own pitch in Connolly Park, Tralee on Saturday, 1st August 2020.

Our game against Kilcummin in Connolly Park was played in dreadful weather conditions on Saturday evening, 1st August 2020. Heavy rain fell all afternoon and persisted right up to half-time in a low scoring game. Despite the inclement weather it was a very enjoyable game and both teams deserved great credit for their efforts. It was a very close game but we finished strongly to win by that most precarious of margins, two points. Final score was 2-5 to 1-6 in favour of Austin Stacks. We now had three points from two games with our third-round game against Killarney Legion fixed for their home pitch at Direen, Killarney on Saturday, 8th August 2020. When word filtered through that Dingle had won their second-round game against Legion it meant that Dingle also had three points with one game each to play. By a strange coincidence, Austin Stacks and Dingle had a similar aggregate score difference so it would be all to play for in Killarney on the following Saturday.

On a beautiful sunny day, which was ideal for playing football, we made the short trip to Direen, Killarney to take on the home team, Killarney Legion. In addition to needing the points and chalking up a better score difference than Dingle in the other game, there was an added dimension to this game. Stephen Stack, who had managed Austin Stacks to Senior County Championship success in 2014 was now managing the Legion. The Rock supporters have great affection for Stephen and are very grateful to him for the success he brought to our club. But today he would be kissing the Legion crest and I was hoping that emotions on both sides would be kept in check. Personally, I like Stephen and admire his passion for success. Moreover, he lives just down the road from me in Spa village. Stephen's children and my grandchildren attend the same school in the village.

In the event, Austin Stacks had a comprehensive win in the game. The team played superbly and were beginning to look like a formidable outfit now that most of our injured players were back to full fitness. Austin Stacks carried the day on a 2-13 to 0-8 scoreline. The big score also put us on top of the table, thus qualifying Austin Stacks for the Senior Club Final against Kenmare Shamrocks. However, before that final would be played another big fixture was beginning to loom large. When I addressed the players after the Legion game to congratulate them on a great win which qualified us for the Senior Club final, I reminded them that we had a date with destiny fast approaching. We were now about to face our biggest challenge of the year against Doctor Crokes, Killarney in the first round of the Kerry Senior Football Championship at Austin Stack Park, Tralee on Friday evening, 21st August 2020, now less than two weeks away. I told the players that they were playing their best football of the season and that I had full confidence in their ability to defeat Doctor Crokes.

There was an eerie atmosphere in an almost empty stadium in Tralee on the evening of the big game. While, I was pleased for our unavoidably absent supporters that TG4 was televising the game live, I was concerned about the absence from the terrace of our famous Rockie supporters who, time and time again, made the difference between a win and a loss. I also felt that the pandemic protocols, the very large stewarding cohort, the distraction of the TG4 crew in the empty venue were very intrusive and unhelpful for the players. I accepted that desperate measures were necessary in desperate times but this was a game I badly wanted to win. Austin Stacks had a superb panel of players. They were good enough to go all the way in this blue riband competition. Before I became Club Chairman in December 2019, I had already prepared a three-year plan leading to County Senior Football Championship success in the third year. I was beginning to revise that plan in my mind on the basis of our talented senior squad, which was playing superb football.

This winner-takes-all-game in Austin Stack Park on the evening of the 21st August 2020 was an emotional roller coaster from start to finish. For those of us who had a stake in the game, it was nerve wracking from the throw in. The teams were level at half time with 1-5 each. At the end of normal time, the team were still level on a score of 2-12 each. When the referee blew the whistle at half time in extra time Doctor Crokes were one point ahead on a scoreline of 2-16 to 2-15. But in the second half of that extra-time, they outscored us by 1-3 to 0-2 to give them a five-points win at the end. The final score was 3-19 to 2-17 in favour of Doctor Crokes.

Austin Stacks had been eliminated from the County Senior Football Championship at the first hurdle. Because of the pandemic, there was to be no losers round in 2020. My ambition to lead The Rock to the Holy Grail in 2020 died a death in a lonely stadium on that fateful Friday night, 21st August 2020. I knew it was my duty as Club Chairman to pick up the players and mentors. There was little or no time for them to feel sorry for themselves or to dwell on the what should have or what could have happened. It was time to focus on the immediate future. In my address, I congratulated the players for a superb effort. They left everything on the field and we were well in the game until Crokes scored a second penalty in the early minutes of the second half of extra time. The Rock team fought to the bitter end. I was very proud of their collective efforts.

I reminded them that we had a prestigious final coming up on the 13th September 2020, when we were scheduled to meet Kenmare Shamrock in the Senior Club final. I asked them to make up for the Senior County Championship elimination by retaining that title which they had won the previous year. I knew the players would need a day or two to shake off the disappointment of the loss to Doctor Crokes, but I knew they had character and were made of stern stuff.

The County Senior Club Final was played in Fitzgerald Stadium Killarney on Sunday afternoon, 13th September, 2020. Once again, the prevailing pandemic regulations meant that attendance was limited and almost unnoticed in the magnificent stadium. It was a very close game where our team had to work very hard to stay in the game. On this occasion, the force was with us and we scored the crucial goal at the right time. The sides were level at five points apiece at the interval break. While Austin Stacks scored the first point of the second half, Kenmare Shamrocks replied with 1-3 to build up a five-point lead as we approached the last five minutes of the game. Deep into injure time the deficit had been reduced to a single goal when, who else but Kieran Donaghy, sent Seán Quilter through for a goal to level matters at 1-9 apiece and send the game into extra time.

Kenmare shaded the first period of extra time by three points to our two to lead by 1-12 to 1-11 going into the second period of extra time. Austin Stacks wasn't about to lose a second consecutive game in extra time and played their best football to outscore Kenmare Shamrocks by six points to two. Austin Stacks were Senior Club Champions for the second year in a row on a scoreline of 1-17 to 1-14. I was delighted for the players and mentors. I thought of our loyal supporters who would love to have shared in the celebrations but were prevented from attending. Celebrations in Tralee would also be curtailed by the restrictions. Since the restrictions had been enforced by the GAA at the beginning of the pandemic, everybody in our club had willingly complied in the interest of public health. I trusted the team management and players to be equally disciplined on Sunday night. Austin Stacks were now holders of the Senior Club trophy and the Senior County League, Division One trophy, which the club had won on the day of my election as Club Chairman on Sunday, 15th December 2019. I knew that my stewardship of Austin Stacks would be remembered not for my administration and restructuring skills but for the number of senior football trophies I delivered. The Rockies have an insatiable appetite for silverware and I fully intended to deliver more during my term of office!

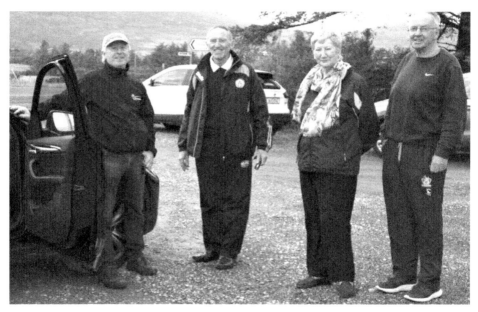

Pictured in Aunnascaul for the Austin Stacks V Dingle game in the Senior Club Championship on the 25th July 2020 were, from left, Éamonn O'Reilly, Billy Ryle, Mairéad Fernane and Colm Mangan

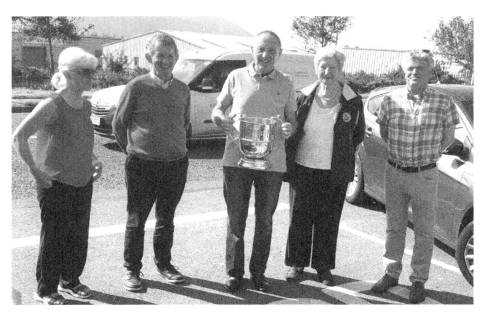

Austin Stacks won the Kerry Senior Club Championship title in Killarney on Sunday, 13th September 2020. Pictured with the Cup are, from left, Liz O'Regan, Nial Shanahan, Billy Ryle, Mairéad Fernane and Denis O'Regan

CHAPTER NINETEEN

WALK THE WALK

On Sunday, 27th September 2020, Austin Stacks captured more silverware by defeating local rivals, John Mitchels in the final of the Tralee District Board Senior Football Championship at Austin Stacks Park, Tralee. The previous weekend, Austin Stacks and John Mitchels had seen off Ballymacelligott and Kerins O'Rahillys, respectively in the semi-finals of that competition. After two hectic games in the County and Club Championships, I would not have been surprised if our boys were feeling tired or lacking in enthusiasm for the game. Not at all, they treated the game very seriously and showed great respect for the competition and the wonderful footballer, the late Roddy O'Donnell, after whom the trophy is named. In addition, the competition is sponsored by Lee Strand Creameries, with which industry the club has a strong association. There was little to separate the sides during the first quarter, with Mitchels having a slight advantage of 1-4 to our 1-3 at the first water break. We just edged the second quarter by one point to leave the sides level at 1-6 apiece at halftime. It was tit-for-tat in the third quarter with our team leading by 1-11 to 2-7 at the second water break. The lead changed again in the final quarter when John Mitchels scored their third goal of the game in the 52nd minute. But their lead was short lived as Austin Stacks scored a goal from the penalty spot. We now had the lead and just about deserved to win by 2-15 to 3-9.

That was our last senior game of the year as Covid-19 had put paid to the Munster and All Ireland Club Championships, both of which competitions we could have won. It wasn't meant to be in 2020. Still and all, after only nine months as Austin Stacks Chairman, we held three major senior trophies – County League and Club Championships and now the Tralee District Board Senior Football Championship. The 'delivery man' had delivered three trophies in his first year as Chairman, but I was very disappointed by our elimination in round one of the County Senior Football Championship. I made a promise to myself that that would never again happen under my watch and I took appropriate action to make sure it didn't.

One of my favourite events on the club's social calendar is the annual Paul Lucey Run/Walk 10k/5k. Because the Covid-19 Pandemic brought our usual fundraising activities to a standstill, the event had more significance than ever in 2020. We decided to hold it virtually to generate badly needed income for the running and upkeep of the Austin Stacks Club and facilities. The Run/Walk on this occasion could be completed, anywhere in the world, in a twenty-four-hour window over the Halloween weekend, Saturday/Sunday, October 31st/Sunday November 1st 2020. Paul was an outstanding clubman who gave sterling service as a player and team manager. The annual 'Run for the Rock' creates a great buzz in the club forecourt before and after the walk and people of all ages enjoy the run or the walk depending on their level of fitness. The social dimension would, of course, be missed in 2020 but we knew that many of our members and supporters were keen to pay tribute to Paul, who is fondly remembered by one and all.

I really enjoyed my own 5km virtual walk in the Paul Lucey Virtual Run/Walk 10k/5k on Sunday morning, 1st November. I followed the same route as in the previous years, from Austin Stack Club entrance gates via Connolly Park turning right into Rock St., then via Stacks Villas onto Caherslee up to Mounthawk Roundabout, turning right into Bracker O'Regan Road, turning right again into Tralee/Fenit greenway and back to Austin Stack Club entrance gates. Jim and Joan Naughton, Colm Mangan, Aoife O' Connell, Pat and Grace Reidy shortened my journey where it felt good to be on the move. Not even the rain could dampen our spirits due to the craic and the banter. We passed a lot of Rockies doing their own virtual run or walk. I was very grateful to everybody who made such a huge effort to honour our great friend, Paul Lucey. Once again, Paul's son, Niall Lucey and his organising team did a marvellous job of providing us with this wonderful annual event while complying with social distancing regulations. If my memory is accurate, the proceeds were used to install single cubicle showers for our lady members. Paul would have been pleased about that as he wanted the best facilities for all of our members, whether female or male.

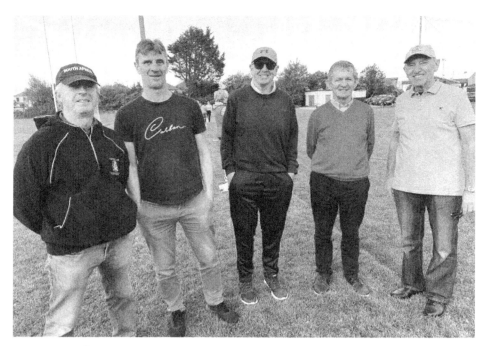

From left, Éamonn O'Reilly, Mike Casey, Colm Mangan, Nial Shanahan and Billy Ryle attended the Austin Stacks v John Mitchels semi-final clash in the Tralee District Senior Football League on the 19th September 2020

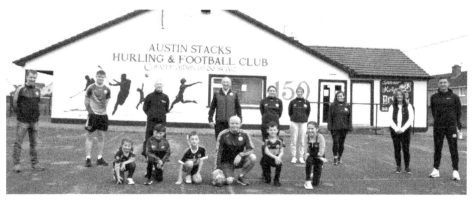

Niall Lucey, front centre, launched the Paul Lucey Memorial 'Run for the Rock' at the Austin Stacks Club Grounds on the 11th October 2020.

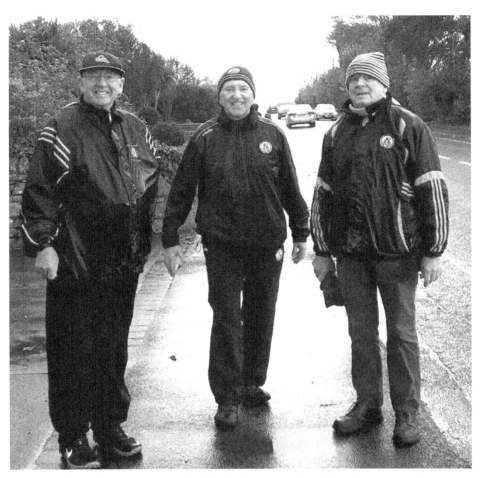

From left, Colm Mangan, Billy Ryle and Jim Naughton on the move during the virtual 'Run for the Rock' on the 1st November 2020

CHAPTER TWENTY

1920 COMMEMORATION CEREMONY

One of the events which made a lasting impression on me was Austin Stack's dignified commemoration of the victims of Bloody Sunday, which was held in the club forecourt on Saturday, 21st November 2020. Because of the Level Five pandemic restrictions that applied at the time, the ceremony was held out of doors and the club membership was represented by a limited number of senior members, including Éamonn O'Reilly, Club Vice Chairman, himself a Tipperary man, Mairéad Fernane, former Club Chairperson, Eddie Barrett, Co. Board Delegate and a grand nephew of the patriot Austin Stack, Jim Naughton, Chairman of the Field Committee, Adrienne McLoughlin, Club Photographer, Carmel Quilter O'Neill, John Breen, Tim Guiheen and myself, Club Chairman. Mairéad, who was the current Oifigeach na Gaeilge agus an Chultúir – Officer for the Irish language and culture - did a great deal of the organisational work for this event. It was very tastefully done. I felt that it was an appropriate and solemn way to remember and honour the fourteen people who lost their lives on that fateful day in Croke Park on Sunday, 21st November 1920. It was my responsibility to deliver the Bloody Sunday Chairman's Oration and I was very honoured to do so. It was an oration for which I did a considerable amount of research and put a considerable amount of thought into. I was determined to deliver an oration which commemorated those who had been killed but to do so in a speech which was built on dignity and reconciliation. The oration follows below.

"A Chairde,
On 21st November 1920, the senior footballers of Dublin and Tipperary were playing a football match in Croke Park when the stadium was invaded by the forces of the British Crown - Army, Royal Irish Constabulary (RIC), Black & Tans and Auxiliaries. With no provocation what-so-ever the British forces indiscriminately opened fire on the

158

crowd. Fourteen innocent men, women and children were killed in that shameful incident. So, tonight, Saturday, 21st November 2020, exactly one hundred years after that infamous episode in the dishonourable history of British imperialism in Ireland, Austin Stacks GAA Club has gathered in the forecourt of our Club facilities and placed fourteen candles, in proud and loving memory of Jane Doyle (26yrs), James Burke (44yrs), Daniel Carroll (31yrs), Michael Ferry (40yrs), Tom Hogan (19yrs), James Matthews (38yrs), Patrick O'Dowd (57yrs), Joe Traynor (21yrs), Jerome O'Leary (10yrs), William Robinson (11yrs), Tom Ryan (27yrs), John William Scott (14yrs), James Teehan (26yrs) and Michael Hogan (24yrs), who lost their lives a century ago. Michael 'Mick' Hogan, after whom The Hogan Stand in Croke Park is named, was corner back on the Tipperary team on that awful day. He was shot in the back as he ran for safety off the pitch. Mick Hogan was the only player killed in Croke Park on Bloody Sunday. The other thirteen were spectators at the match. More than sixty-five people were also injured, some seriously.

My gratitude to Club Vice Chairman, Éamonn O Reilly, a Tipperary native, for presenting us with a replica of the jersey worn by Mick Hogan and his Tipperary team mates on that fateful afternoon. The jersey is proudly on display here this evening alongside our own black and amber flag as a gesture of solidarity with the Tipperary and Dublin footballers of 1920. No doubt, Éamonn is hoping that the jersey will bring Tipperary success over Cork in tomorrow's Munster Senior Football Championship Final!

On this centenary milestone, we also fondly remember the members of the fledgling Rock Street Club who suffered and died during the War of Independence. Some of those patriots had helped to established the Rock Street Club in 1917 to promote Gaelic games and to oppose all things British. They were the people who set the standards, aims and values that the Austin Stack Club continues to champion to this very day. They are all in our thoughts and prayers on this solemn occasion. On 5th January 1933, the Rock Street Club, which has deep roots embedded in the cause of Irish freedom, was renamed The Austin Stacks Hurling and Football Club in honour of the great Irish Patriot, Austin

Stack. Eddie Barrett, a grand-nephew of Austin Stack is one of the people representing our Club here this evening. Eddie is a life-long and committed activist in the Rock Club. It's well worth remembering that, during the height of the War of Independence and in very difficult circumstances, The Rock managed to field a team which won the Kerry Junior Football Championship in 1921, just four years after its founding. This title is very precious. It was achieved without the services of a number of Rock Street Republicans who were on the run, interned or imprisoned. It was the first of the Clubs many subsequent successes. It is my sincere hope, and it would be entirely appropriate, that Austin Stacks should win the Kerry Senior Football Championship in 2021, a hundred years after its first county title success."

Mairéad Fernane, Irish language and culture Officer in the Austin Stack Club, my predecessor as Club Chairperson and a niece of Big Dan O Sullivan, our first Chairman in 1917, then led us in a decade of the Rosary for the happy repose of the souls of the fourteen innocent people who left home on Sunday, 21st November 1920 to attend a football match in Croke Park but never returned. Mairéad then followed the prayers with a rendition of our Club Anthem, 'The Boys from the top of the Rock.

The Boys from the top of the Rock
By
Ned Drummond

If you want to be happy the rest of your life
Come up to the top of the Rock
It's the grandest spot in Ireland
And full of the rare auld stock
No matter what your past may be
If you haven't the price of a block
They'll never see you down and out
Above at the top of the Rock.

Our glorious Gaelic footballers are champions of Tralee
They've beaten all before them
From Strand Road to Boherbee
Purty plays full-forward
And Barrett stands the shock
You can back your bottom dollar
On the boys from the top of the Rock

Our sporty men of different shades
Their equals can't be found
Lovers of the feathered race
The horse, the rod and hound.
You have Rory O'Connell's Fanbelt
And Paddy Casey's gamecock
Bred, born and reared
Above at the top of the Rock

Pádraig Mac Piarais designated the beautiful Irish ballad, 'Óró sé do bheatha bhaile' as the marching song of the Easter Rising. It was also retained as the marching song of the Irish Volunteers in the War of Independence. I led those present in singing a rousing rendition of that song to bring the Blood Sunday Commemoration Ceremony to a fitting conclusion.

Oró, Sé Do Bheatha 'Bhaile/Oh-ro, welcome home

By

Unknown Author & Pádraig Mac Piarais

Óró 'Sé do bheatha 'bhaile, / Oh-ro, welcome home,
Óró 'Sé do bheatha 'bhaile, / Oh-ro, welcome home,
Óró 'Sé do bheatha 'bhaile, / Oh-ro, welcome home,
Anois ar theacht an tsamhraidh! / Now that summer's coming!

'Sé do bheatha a bhean ba léanmhar, / Hail, oh woman, who was so
afflicted,
B' é ár gcreach tú bheith i ngéibhinn, / It was our ruin that you were in
chains,
Do dhúiche bhreá i seilibh meirleach, / Our fine land in the possession
of thieves,
Is tú díolta leis na Gallaibh! / While you were sold to the foreigners!

Óró 'Sé do bheatha 'bhaile,
Óró 'Sé do bheatha 'bhaile,
Óró 'Sé do bheatha 'bhaile,
Anois ar theacht an tsamhraidh!

Tá Gráinne Mhaol ag teacht thar sáile, / Gráinne Mhaol is coming over
the sea,
Óglaigh armtha léi mar gharda, / Armed warriors as her guard,
Gaeil iad féin is ní Gaill ná Spáinnigh / Only Gaels are they, not French
nor Spanish,
Is cuirfidh siad ruaig ar Ghallaibh! / And they will rout the foreigners!

Óró 'Sé do bheatha 'bhaile,
Óró 'Sé do bheatha 'bhaile,
Óró 'Sé do bheatha 'bhaile,
Anois ar theacht an tsamhraidh!

A bhuí le Rí na bhFeart go bhfeiceann, / May it please the King of
Prodigy that we might see,

Muna mbíonn beo ina dhiaidh ach seachtain, / Although we may live but one week after,
Gráinne Mhaol is míle gaiscíoch / Gráinne Mhaol and a thousand warriors,
Ag fógairt fáin ar Ghallaibh! / Dispersing the foreigners!

Óró 'Sé do bheatha 'bhaile,
Óró 'Sé do bheatha 'bhaile,
Óró 'Sé do bheatha 'bhaile,
Anois ar theacht an tsamhraidh!

When I mentioned in my oration that in 2021 it would be one hundred years since Austin Stacks, then called Rock Street, had won a County Championship title for the first time, I felt a positive karma descending on me. It's difficult to put these warm feelings into words, but I somehow knew that 2021 would be a successful year for Austin Stacks. I am a spiritual person, who in a forecourt with a small number of colleagues on a dark winter's night, felt the presence of the ghosts of over a century of our deceased members. Was I imagining things or was 2021 going to be the year when The Bishop Moynihan trophy would finally return to The Rock?

 Mairéad Fernane's exceptional organisational skills were seen at their best at the poignant commemoration. Her thoughtfulness at displaying fourteen candles, one representing each of the fourteen people who were killed, brought a tear to my eye. In keeping with the national mood of solemnity and remembrance of those dark events a century ago, club members honoured the fourteen victims of Bloody Sunday in 1920 by lighting a candle for each of the dead. The tiny flicker of candle light that withstood a dark and chilly November evening at Austin Stacks GAA Club grounds set the reverent atmosphere and helped to revive one of Irish history's bleakest moments. It was also a great privilege to receive from Club Vice-Chairman Éamonn O'Reilly - a Tipperary native - a replica of the jersey worn by Michael Hogan and his Tipperary team mates on that fateful afternoon in 1920. It's a commemoration that I will always remember.

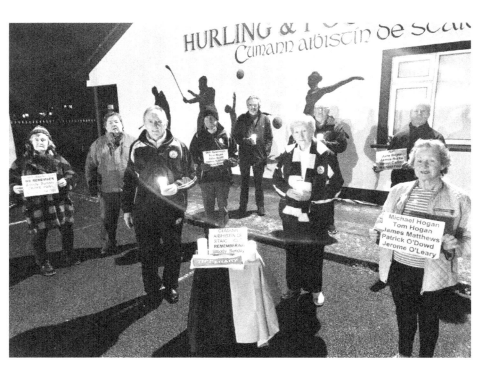

Austin Stacks GAA Club commemorated 'Bloody Sunday 1920' with a dignified ceremony at the Club's Grounds, Connolly Park, Tralee on the 21st November 2020. Pictured L/r: Adrienne McLoughlin, Eddie Barrett, Billy Ryle, Jim Naughton, John Breen, Mairéad Fernane, Tim Guiheen, Éamonn O'Reilly and Carmel Quilter O'Neill

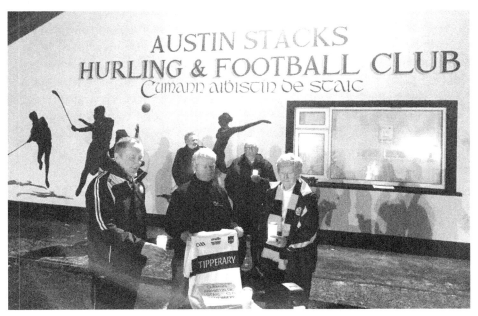

Éamonn O'Reilly, Austin Stacks Vice-Chairman and a Tipperary man, displays a replica of the jersey worn by the Tipperary team in Croke Park on Bloody Sunday 1920. Pictured, from left, Billy Ryle, Club Chairman, John Breen, Éamonn O'Reilly, Tim Guiheen and Mairéad Fernane, former Chairperson at the Austin Stacks 'Bloody Sunday 1920' commemoration service on the 21st November 2020

CHAPTER TWENTY ONE

CONSIDERING A CORNEAL TRANSPLANT

It was now almost six months since I last had an appointment with Mr Flynn, so I was looking forward to my appointment with him at The Elysian in Cork on the 27th November 2020. It was now coming up to the first anniversary of the cataract surgery which I underwent at Bon Secours Hospital, Cork in December 2019. I was so busy in my role of Austin Stacks Chairman and the great difficulties caused by the Covid-19 pandemic that I had little time to dwell on the problem with my eyes. I had developed a number of coping strategies such as reading books with enlarged print, driving locally only and wearing sunglasses where ever possible, particularly when I was gardening or painting or doing routine maintenance around the house.

Mister Flynn felt that the vision in my right eye had not improved much since the cataract surgery. There had been a minor improvement from wearing the new glasses. Mister Flynn assured me that the eye appeared healthy apart from diffuse corneal thickening due to the Fuchs Dystrophy. He said it was now reasonable to consider a corneal endothelial graft to improve vision. He provided me with printed information on the procedure and explained that it may need more than one operation as 20% need repeat gas tamponade to optimise graft attachment. He told me that I would have to make several visits to the clinic and use eyedrops for at least a year. Mr Flynn said that there was a very good chance of improving the vision and a small chance of making the vision worse. He requested me to study the information and he said he would see me again in the New Year to make a decision on the corneal transplant. I found his directness very refreshing. He spelt out very clearly that there were risks attached to the surgery and there was a possibility of my sight being worse afterwards. At this stage, having been his patient for a year, I had complete and total confidence in Mr Flynn's judgement and I was more than happy to have the transplant surgery. However, I knew it wouldn't go ahead until Mr Flynn felt it was the right time to operate. Twelve months earlier, I thought I would be done and dusted in a year. Now I knew exactly how serious by eyes' condition was. I had a disease that had to be monitored but the timing of the surgical procedures needed to counteract it would be determined by the deterioration of the cornea. I needed to be patient and let nature takes its course. I accepted that I would be making frequent visits to Cork and could expect at least three more visits as a patient to the Bon Secours Hospital in College Road. In the meantime, I would read the literature in order to learn as much as possible about a corneal transplant. On my way out, the Practice Co-Ordinator fixed my next appointment with Mr Flynn for the 23rd February 2021. I had high hopes that in 2021 further progress would be made with the problems in my eyes. Having come this far, I was determined to do what I needed to do to solve the problem. I felt it would be well worth the effort if I regained a quality of vision that would keep me functioning independently for the remainder of my life.

As I journeyed home on the train, I convinced myself that I had little to complain about. I had managed fairly comfortably during the past year. While the cataract surgery hadn't resulted in any significant improvement in the vision in my right eye, neither had there been any noticeable deterioration. From travelling up and down to Cork during the past year, I learned for a fact that there were many people visiting consultants with medical conditions that were far more serious than mine.

I was delighted by the wonderful news on Christmas Eve that An Bord Pleanála had granted planning permission to Fenit Development Association for the new diving boards at the bathing slip. In arriving at its decision to grant permission for the project, An Bord Pleanála took the Kerry County Development Plan into consideration to facilitate the development of sustainable water sports. It had been a long and difficult campaign since 2017 and the positive outcome was a tribute to my colleagues, Mike O Neill, Liam Doyle, Paddy Kissane and John Edwards for their vision, altruism and determination to bring this wonderful public project to the crucial stage of planning approval.

I missed the traditional buzz, atmosphere, razzamatazz and craic of the cancelled midday swim in Fenit on Christmas Day, 2020 but the decision not to go ahead with a mass swim was the correct one for public health reasons. The picturesque village of Fenit annually hosts the best attended Christmas swim in Ireland.

The very first Christmas Day swim in Fenit took place on 25th December 1952 just six months after Tralee Swimming Club was founded at a meeting in The Grand Hotel, Denny Street on the 21st June 1952, the summer solstice, which was a most appropriate day to found a swimming club. Connie Foley, 'The Whistling Postman' became the first Chairman of Tralee Swimming Club.

PJ Costello is the only surviving member of the group which took part in the first Christmas Day swim at the bathing slip. The others present at the swim were Michael O' Regan, Pat Hickey, Connie Foley, Paddy O'Sullivan, Fionán Harty, Gerald Walsh, Tom Reidy and Michael Morris. The Christmas swim has grown in stature to a proportion which this pioneering group could hardly have imagined on an inclement and blustery Christmas morning in 1952.

Nowadays, about 2,000 people flock to the seaside village of Fenit from 11am on Christmas morning to participate in a memorable annual event. Half of them take the plunge into the cold sea while the remainder enjoy the spectacle from the relative comfort of dry land. Not so in 2020 but, please God, there would be many more Christmas day swims.

For my swim on Christmas Day 2020, instead of charging to the ocean in the midst of a crowd, I enjoyed a relaxed afternoon dip at the bathing slip in Fenit to whet the appetite for the Christmas dinner and to maintain my tradition of a Christmas plunge. It was lovely to see people taking a stroll or a dip while observing social distancing and complying with the NPHET protocols.

The swim itself was a spiritual experience, reminding me of the fragility of life and nature. I have always taken the swim for granted as part of my Christmas day routine. However, the pandemic had taught me to ground myself in the moment and live each day to the full within the restrictions that applied at the time. As one accustomed to swimming in choppy waters, I dedicated my Christmas dip in 2020 to Dr Tony Holohan, a selfless national hero, who was currently swimming against a very strong tide. But even the highest tide must turn and I was confident that Dr Holohan would lead us safely ashore if we followed his firm strokes.

CHAPTER TWENTY TWO

UNDERSTANDING CORNEAL SURGERY

In the expectation that I would surely have a corneal transplant of a donor organ in one eye, if not both, during 2021, I spent the Christmas period reading through the information that Mr Flynn had given me about corneal transplantation.

I learned that the cornea is a window of transparent tissue at the front of the eyeball. It allows light to pass into the eye and provides focus so that images can be seen. Various diseases or injury can make the cornea either cloudy or out of shape. This prevents the normal passage of light and affects vision. The cornea has three layers – thin outer and inner layers and a thick middle layer. In some diseases, only the inside layer, called Endothelium, is affected. This causes swelling and clouding. Endothelial Keratoplasty is a modern technique to replace the inside layer of the cornea with the inside layer from a donor cornea through a relatively small incision, restoring clarity whilst leaving the healthy parts of the cornea unaltered. This procedure usually has a relatively faster recovery rate and a lower rejection rate than the alternative procedure where a layer of cells is transplanted along with a slice of supporting tissue from the back of the donor cornea.

As is the case with most medical procedures, there are benefits and risks associated with Endothelial Keratoplasty. The obvious benefit is improved vision. 80% of transplant recipients reach driving standard if the eye is otherwise healthy but may need glasses. It may take up to six months until the full improvement is appreciated. Comfort is improved in some cases. The risks associated with Endothelial Keratoplasty can be categorised as follows.

1 Rare but serious complications

- Sight-threatening infection in one in five hundred cases

- Severe haemorrhage causing loss of vision
- Retinal detachment

2 Corneal transplant rejection

- A corneal transplant can be identified and attacked by your immune system. This happens in a low percentage of recipients in the first two years after transplantation and can cause graft failure. It can often be reversed if anti-rejection medication is started promptly. Rejection remains a possibility for your lifetime.

3 Graft Failure

- When a graft fails the cornea becomes cloudy again and vision becomes blurred

4 Glaucoma

- This can usually be controlled by eyedrops but occasionally requires surgery

5 Graft Dislocation

- About 20% of Endothelial Keratoplasty grafts dislocate in the days or weeks after surgery and need to be repositioned by an air or gas injection in the eye. This can be carried out either in theatre or in clinic.

6 Cataract

- This can be removed surgically

Endothelial Keratoplasty has a number of possible advantages over full-thickness graft. The recovery time is faster. There are less stitches used which means that the shape of the cornea is more normal and the patient is less dependent on glasses or contact lens. The wound is smaller so fewer wound complications such as leakage or traumatic wound rupture are likely to occur. There is also a lower risk of the recipient's immune system damaging the graft.

The Operation

The operation is performed under local anaesthetic and takes about one hour. Through a small incision the patient's endothelium is removed and a disc of donor endothelium is inserted and pressed in position against the back of the patient's cornea by a bubble of air or gas. You may be asked to lie flat for one or two hours after the operation. One or two stitches in the cornea are often used. These are easily removed in the weeks after surgery.

After the Operation

You will be examined by Mr Flynn after the surgery and usually stay in hospital for one night. You can usually go home the next day. You will be seen again within one week to access whether the graft has stayed in position. You will have about six visits to the outpatient clinic in the first year. It is generally recommended that you take two weeks off work. You will need to use anti-rejection eyedrops for at least twelve months and in some cases indefinitely. The stitches are usually removed about one month after the operation.

What if the transplant fails?

- A failed transplant can be replaced in a procedure known as a regraft.

Corneal Transplant Rejection

- If this is not treated urgently it can lead to failure of the transplant and loss of vision.

Symptoms of Rejection

- Red eye
- Sensitivity to light
- Visual loss
- Pain

I studied the literature very carefully and while I couldn't admit to understanding all of the medical terminology, I was left in no doubt that this was a very serious operation which would only go ahead under ideal conditions. It was up to me to avoid illness of any kind and to remain healthy. With the country ravaged by the pandemic and the flu bug, I made a determined effort to isolate and to avoid situations where I might be at risk. I made sure that I took the vaccine when I was required to do so. I kept up my fitness with regular walking and swimming.

I was aware that I would receive a donor organ. The person donating the cornea would have died but would have willed that the organ, and possibly other organs, be given to a person like myself who needed it. It was an altruistic gesture by the anonymous individual concerned. The donors were in my thoughts and prayers.

The main post-operative risks were infection and rejection of the organ. I knew I was disciplined enough to follow the instructions in the literature as I was determined that all would turn out well. It was a waiting game now but I began to notice that my eyesight was beginning to slowly but gradually deteriorate.

CHAPTER TWENTY THREE

PUBLIC HEALTH GUIDELINES

As the new year of 2021 was being heralded in, I felt it necessary as Chairman of Austin Stacks to issue a fresh appeal to our members to continue complying with the public health guidelines in the commendable manner in which they had done so in 2020. I was very proud of the Club's united effort and solidarity in that regard in 2020. I regretted than many of them were unable to attend our matches, but I knew that they took some solace from the successful year we had on the field. We had the Senior Club and Senior League trophies in our possession but I was very disappointed by our early exit from the County Senior Championship. My appeal was circulated through all of our media outlets as I wanted all arteries of the club to be fully conversant with my strategy for the months ahead. In my appeal, I said that last March, I requested all members of our Club to comply fully with the GAA and the Government national public health guidelines against the coronavirus pandemic.

"Our Club rose to the challenge and played its part in the battle against this deadly Covid-19 virus. As well as that, the Austin Stacks GAA Club Community Response to helping those in need showed the true character of the Club. Our entire membership showed great restraint in complying with the safety regulations. The discipline, solidarity and high standards shown by our members reflected our core values. Unfortunately, the virus is again all pervasive and I must, once again, request all members of Austin Stacks to comply with the recently issued GAA and Government guidelines, which are in place until the 31st January, at least. The Club specific guidelines issued by the GAA are as follows. In Level Five, individual training only is permitted. Neither adult nor underage teams may train collectively. GAA club grounds must stay closed. Club games are not permitted. Dressing rooms, showers and all other indoor training facilities must remain closed for club activities. Club Gyms must remain closed until further notice. No indoor meetings can be held. All officer training must be delivered online. Outdoor coaching education courses are not permitted. Club Bars must remain closed until the current restrictions are lifted. No organised indoor gatherings can take place under the current restrictions. Commercial use of indoor halls, for example by state bodies– e.g., HSE/Schools, is permitted where agreement was in place prior to last March and relevant insurances are in place. These are the only instances in which indoor activity is permitted on GAA Club property. No outdoor gatherings on GAA property are permitted. Please stay safe and avoid any breach of the regulations that could place yourself or any club colleagues or, indeed the public at large in danger of contracting the coronavirus. I assure you that we will get the training and games up and running for the sake of player mental health, welfare and wellbeing, as soon as it's safe to do so. All social activity in the Club will resume when we are permitted to do so," I added.

In the meantime, our Juvenile Club and Senior Club Annual General Meetings were on the horizon. Unfortunately, it wasn't possible to have the AGMs in person so we went virtual on the Microsoft Teams platform. I'm very much a face-to-face communicator, who likes to establish a good rapport based on a friendly, harmonious relationship, characterized by agreement, mutual understanding and empathy that makes communication easier. I've always regarded body language an integral component of effective communication. In addition, the virtual meetings were a new and unfamiliar departure for me. Chairing a meeting while manipulating the various functions of the platform was going to be a huge challenge for me. Tim McMahon, Chairman of our Juvenile Club would be in the hot seat for the Juvenile AGM and I was hoping to pick up the technique from him. In preparing my address, I deliberately concentrated on updating the attendance on club policy and outlining the importance of the great work they do with our young members.

I began by thanking Juvenile Chairman, Tim McMahon for the invitation to join the Juvenile Club AGM and I said that I was delighted with the opportunity to share some information with those in attendance.

"It's been a very difficult year for sport, not only for our own club but for sports clubs in general. Just when our playing season was getting into full swing, it was abruptly halted by the coronavirus pandemic and never really recovered. Our young members have suffered a torrid time since, being denied the joy of training and the thrill of competition. They have missed out on many of the activities that young people normally take for granted. Their mental health has been challenged, their ability to cope has been severely tested and their way of life has been cruelly interrupted.

Last March, I requested all units of our club to comply fully with the GAA and the Government public health guidelines. Austin Stacks rose to the challenge and played its part in the battle against this deadly Covid-19 virus. As well as that, the Austin Stacks GAA Club Community Response to helping those in need showed the true character of the club. Our administrators and team mentors can be particularly proud of their leadership during the year. The discipline, solidarity and high standards shown by our members reflected our core values. Unfortunately, the virus has lingered and I am obliged to again request all club members to comply with GAA and Government public health guidelines for as long as is necessary. How long the restrictions are going to last is anybody's guess but I assure you we will get the training and games up and running for the sake of player mental health, welfare and wellbeing, as soon as it's safe to do so.

Éamonn O'Reilly, Club Vice Chairman and myself, with invaluable assistance from Eddie Barrett and Shane Lynch made a determined effort last year to source sponsorship. We were anxious that none of our activities would be curtailed by lack of funding. I'm glad to report that we have been fairly successful in our efforts. Kirby's Brogue Inn and Restaurant came on board as our main sponsors for a three-year period beginning in 2020. I'm delighted that our senior team delivered the Kerry Senior Club Championship and the Tralee District Board Championship to repay The Brogue's support of Austin Stacks. Ross Jewellers donated €1000 which was spent on three sets of Juvenile jerseys. I'm delighted to inform you this evening that Ned O'Shea Construction and Lane Food Distributors have agreed to jointly provide a three-year sponsorship for our Juvenile Club from 2021. I intend that the money provided will be used in its entirety to cover juvenile costs. The incoming Club Executive will meet on 20th January 2021 and Tim will report back to you with the up-to-date details.

I firmly believe that clear and effective up and down communication throughout our club is vital for good management. It means we are all well informed about club policy and issues that may arise from time to time. My chairmanship of Austin Stacks is based on openness, democracy and inclusion. The monthly meetings of our Club Executive Committee are very efficient and based on information sharing, open discussion and democratic decision making. I emphasise policy-based discussion, mutual respect and delegation of workload so that no member is overburdened. With that in mind, a number of focussed subcommittees were established last year and they have enriched and concentrated the work that we do.

The Juvenile Club is a very important part of that structure. You have your own juvenile subcommittee or juvenile executive committee, if you'd prefer, which manages under age activities in our club. It's chaired by the Juvenile Club Chairman and I'm fully aware of the great work that you do. Similar to the main Club Executive Committee, I'd encourage your executive to meet on a monthly basis so that we can have direct and immediate feedback in both directions. I'd love, also, if some of you would consider joining any of our subcommittees. For example, your Treasurer would be a great asset on our Finance Committee. Éamonn O'Reilly is Chairman of our Coaching and Games Development subcommittee and he would welcome people with that kind of interest and expertise.

In total, we have seven subcommittees - JobMatch, Field, Social, Finance, Juvenile, Gaeilge/Cultúir, Coaching/Games Development and Lotto - and I'm hoping to set up one or two more on the 20th January. Tim will give you detailed feedback and please consider getting involved in a subcommittee to which you feel you can contribute. Thank you all most sincerely for your generous contribution to Austin Stacks and especially to the young people you work with. You are the people who impart firm values, ambition, a sense of community, a work ethic, good life-skills and a lifelong affection for Austin Stacks to the young people you interact with. You expose the youngsters to the sheer joy of playing games and whatever competitive success it brings. You provide a conveyer belt of footballers, many of whom go on to great things with Austin Stacks and Kerry.

Mar a deireann an seanfhocal, tús maith leath na hoibre – a good start is half the work. All of you are giving the Austin Stacks juveniles the best possible start in life. You can be proud of and take great satisfaction from the wonderful work that you do on behalf of our great Club," I added.

Tim did a great job in his stewardship of the meeting and his efficiency on virtual media was admirable. I was very impressed by the various reports and the positive feedback that followed. It was a very ebullient AGM and I was able to sense the anticipation of the attendance to get back out on the training pitches with their young charges.

CHAPTER TWENTY FOUR

FOCUS ON SENIOR COUNTY CHAMPIONSHIP

The Senior Club Annual General Meeting was fixed for the 13th January 2021. I put a great deal of thought and preparation into my address to the AGM. I outlined the progress made by my Executive Committee and myself during the past year. I was determined to pay well deserved tribute to the extraordinary level of volunteering in the club during 2020. I made a point of acknowledging our successes on the field. Most importantly, I left the meeting in no doubt that I was totally focussed on winning the 2021 County Senior Football Championship. I regretted that the AGM was held virtually as nothing beats an in-person meeting to rally the troops, to soak up the atmosphere and to set out our stall for titles in the year ahead. Nevertheless, the AGM was a great success and twelve months after I had become Chairman, I now felt that I was leading a totally united club.

I told those present that it had been a very difficult year for sports clubs, including our own. Despite the challenges presented by the pandemic, a united and disciplined Austin Stacks Club weathered the storm well. I added that we had complied with all the Government and GAA health directives and emerged stronger than ever.

"Unfortunately, a very virulent strain of the virus is now circulating and we must again comply with GAA and Government public health guidelines for as long as is necessary. How long the lock down will last is anybody's guess. But we will get the training and games up and running for the welfare, wellbeing and mental health of our players, as soon as it's safe to do so. We'll move forward together with the unity, common purpose and the passion for success that makes our club so special.

Despite the restrictions imposed by the pandemic, 2020 was a very progressive year for Austin Stacks both on and off the pitch. We cleared the debt on our second pitch, which we now own outright. We replaced the netting between the pitches and we upgraded the goalposts. We installed new shower units in the Gym which are also suitable for use by Austin Stacks Ladies Club. Our external clubhouse walls were freshly painted by club volunteers and beautifully illustrated by mural artist, Mike O' Donnell. The upgrading of the heating system in our Club Bar and Hall will be completed shortly. We have plans to further enhance our outdoor facilities this year when the season reopens.

Our on-field, activity was considerably curtailed last year. Our players have endured a torrid time, being denied the joy of training and the thrill of competition. They have missed out on many of the activities that players normally take for granted. Their emotional health has been challenged. Their coping skills have been severely tested. Their expectation of a full season was cruelly shattered. I'm very grateful to all our team officials, who did their very best to provide sanctioned activity for the players. We got a most welcome psychological lift from our wonderful Senior A team, which delivered the County Senior Club Championship and the Tralee District Board Championship. Congratulations to the team and mentors for lifting our spirits in a time of need.

There is a perception gaining currency that the Kerry Senior Football Championship will be the preserve of the multi-club Divisional Board teams for the foreseeable future and that long established clubs like Stacks, Kerins O'Rahillys, Doctor Crokes and Legion will have to make do with the support competitions - County League and County Club Championship. Austin Stacks will never subscribe to that tall tale. Austin Stacks aims to win every competition it participates in, including the County Senior Football Championship.

It's well worth recalling that 100yrs ago in very difficult circumstances, the fledgling Rock Street Club managed to field a team which won the Kerry Junior Football Championship, just four years after its founding. That title is very precious to Austin Stacks and the spirit of 1921 will always inspire us. It was achieved without a number of Rock Street Republicans who were on the run, interned or imprisoned. It was the first of the club's many subsequent successes. It's my sincere hope, and it will be entirely appropriate and symbolic, that Austin Stacks will win the 2021 Kerry Senior Football Championship, a hundred years after its first county title success.

Éamonn O'Reilly, Club Vice Chairman and myself, with invaluable assistance from Eddie Barrett and Shane Lynch made a determined effort last year to source sponsorship. We were anxious that none of our activities would be curtailed by lack of funding. We have been fairly successful in our efforts. Kirby's Brogue Inn and Restaurant came on board as our main sponsors for a three-year period beginning in 2020. Ross Jewellers sponsored our u-12 team last year and I'm delighted to inform you that Ned O'Shea Construction and John Lane Wholesale Food Distributors have agreed to jointly provide a three-year sponsorship for our Juvenile Club from 2021. My sincere thanks to all our sponsors and I assure them that we value their financial support for Austin Stacks.

Effective up and down communication throughout our club is one of my key administrative objectives. It's vital for good management and good morale. It means that we are all fully informed about club policy and activities. The monthly meetings of our Club Executive Committee are business-like and productive. We share information. We have open and frank discussion and our decisions are democratically arrived at. Our deliberations are policy driven and our work is shared so that no member is overburdened. With that in mind, eight subcommittees, each chaired by a member of the Executive Committee, were established or reorganised during the past year, namely - JobMatch, Field, Lotto, Social, Finance, Juvenile, Gaeilge/Cultúir and Coaching/Games Development. The excellent contribution of these subcommittees has enhanced the quality of the service provided to our members. We hope to set up one or two more subcommittees in 2021 to complete the efficient administration of the club. All of these subcommittees have a focussed brief and will welcome new members in 2021. The club has many fine members whose expertise will be invaluable on these subcommittees.

Looking ahead to 2021, please stay safe and avoid any breach of the regulations that could place yourself or any club colleagues or, indeed the public at large, in danger of contracting the coronavirus. My priority is to get the training and games up and running as soon as we are given the all clear to do so. Our facilities are missing the buzz of activity created by players enjoying training and games. We have missed the special roar of the Rockies since last March. We are chomping at the bit to resume normal service.

I regret that I was unable last year to call a meeting of hurling enthusiasts in the club because of the lockdown. I'm aware that we have many members who are passionate about hurling so. I assure you that hurling is close to the top of my to-do list in 2021.

As many of you may be aware, Larry McCarthy, Michael Naughton and Hilda Breslin will this year become Presidents, respectively, of the GAA, The Ladies Gaelic Football Association (LGFA) and The Camogie Association. I congratulate all three of them and wish them every success, but I am sending them a clear and unambiguous message from Austin Stacks. End the procrastination that has lingered for far too long. Stop dragging your feet and amalgamate the three bodies under the Gaelic Athletic Association. The people who founded the GAA in Hayes Hotel in Thurles in 1884 would approve of ladies having full and equal status in the GAA. We are now living in an era of liberty, equality and fraternity. Here in Austin Stacks, we have a large and successful Ladies Gaelic Football Club that is valued and admired by all of us. We work as a single unit as far as possible but the fact remains that the Ladies Club is affiliated to the LGFA. The club I chair is affiliated to the GAA. This is a year when some commentators will highlight historical division in our country. But it's also a year when our three associations can unite under the umbrella of the GAA. We're all part of the same Gaelic games' family with the common aim of promoting Gaelic games and Irish culture. There is strength in unity. Together in one association, we will grow stronger with a single administration, the best facilities and a common bond between all members, male and female.

Austin Stacks is famous for its Rockie Army of supporters. We are one of the best supported clubs in the country. I am appealing to every supporter, at home and abroad, to become a club member for 2021. Our fundraising was curtailed in 2020 by the coronavirus. The same is likely to happen this year. So please, if this club means anything to you, don't just be a supporter, but also pay your membership.

All of us who are active in The Rock are doing so in a voluntary capacity. We do it for the great affection we have for Austin Stacks and for the personal satisfaction of contributing to a great club. Volunteers are rarely thanked and often criticised. I want to express my sincere gratitude to every member who has contributed to Austin Stacks in 2020 from our distinguished Club President, Brendan Dowling right through to our most humble and unassuming voluntary worker.

When I addressed our last AGM in December 2019, I told you that my motto as Club Chairman is an adaptation of JFK's motto from his inauguration speech as President of the USA in January,1961. 'Ask not what your club can do for you. Rather ask what you can do for your club.' You responded with generosity in 2020. I am counting on you to do likewise in 2021," I said.

I welcomed the newly elected Executive Committee to its first meeting on the 20th January 2021. I was delighted to have a few new members, as they usually arrive with lots of enthusiasm and energy. New ideas and fresh thinking revitalise any committee. Austin Stacks was blessed with a lovely blend of old and new members who would deliver for the club in 2021. At that stage, Austin Stacks held the Senior Club Championship title and the Senior County League Division One titles. Our senior playing squad was so strong and talented that I was very keen to retain those titles in 2021. I was anxious to supply strong panels also for our Senior B and C squads, The management teams of the Senior B and Senior C teams were very dedicated and I wanted them to have every chance of success in the coming year.

For my Executive and myself, the overriding ambition in 2021 was to win the County Senior Football Championship. This was a title which had eluded the club since our last victory in 2014. The Executive had a detailed discussion about how to go about achieving that aim. Éamonn O'Reilly, Club Vice-Chairman was also our Coaching and Games Development Officer. Éamonn had achieved commendable progress in that portfolio during the past year despite being curtailed by the coronavirus pandemic. He has the extraordinary capacity to get the best out of people. He has a warm non-threatening personality which appeals to people. His plans for coaching and development were warmly received by our club coaches. His views were well considered and delivered with confidence and authority at the Executive meeting. Éamonn had also liaised closely with the senior team management during the year as well as being a member of the Senior B management team. He was a busy man with his finger on the pulse of senior football in the club. I also appreciated his courtesy in regularly keeping me up to speed on all matters on the field.

Decisions were taken which paid rich dividends in the senior competitions that were to come later in the year. Éamonn O' Reilly, Mike Casey, Colm Mangan and Tim McMahon were appointed to maintain a close liaison with the Senior A management team. Mikey Collins, former star footballer, was added to the Senior A management team. Tim McMahon and Mikey Collins were also drafted on to the Senior B management team. A firm commitment was also made to provide every possible support to the personable Aidan O'Connor and his mentors in their efforts to field a strong Senior C team, which was affectionally called "Charlie's Angels" in memory of the late great Charlie Healy.

CHAPTER TWENTY FIVE

GAA DISCIPLINE

I had hoped that Austin Stacks would be able to resume activities in February 2021. That could not happen as the virus was still very virulent. All our facilities would remain in total lockdown until 5th March. As a united club, we had been noble to-date in complying with Government and GAA directives. That had to continue for as long as it took to suppress this dreadful virus. The official position of Austin Stacks GAA Club was that we were in full lockdown and all activities were suspended in line with public health and GAA regulations. Austin Stacks had always promoted high standards, good discipline, unity of purpose and patriotism in the face of a national crisis. Once again, we were wearing the green jersey to combat the coronavirus.

However, I asked all our members via our media outlets to "please keep in mind that, while each one of us must lead by example, at the end of the day we are all volunteers. All breaches of public health regulations and civil law are a matter for An Garda Siochána. As Club Chairman, I feel a strong duty of care for the safety and wellbeing of our entire membership. In the current tense environment, a growing number of people are taking exception to the restrictions. Please do not put your personal safety at risk by confronting trespassers on our pitches or in our buildings. We saw the tragic consequences of a well-meant intervention by a talented young sportsman in Dublin last week. His life was cruelly ended in a matter of seconds."

I fully concurred with outgoing GAA President, John Horan's views that the GAA's reaction to the coronavirus pandemic had served the country well. As he magnanimously offered the use of GAA facilities for the roll-out of vaccines, John added that the GAA should be able to assist Pharmacists and GPs in the roll-out of the vaccine, provided the insurance and safety protocols were in place. He said that if the GAA could do this, as a final act in fighting the virus, it would have served the country well.

John Horan was justifiably scathing of those who breached training bans and match day protocols, insisting they showed a lack of respect for people's health by their actions. While accepting that the number of violations was tiny in the context of overall GAA activity, the President said that it reflected badly on those who led or allowed those breaches of the regulations to happen.

As his term as President of the GAA came to an end, Austin Stacks paid warm tribute to John Horan for his solid and progressive leadership of our Association. We also extended our best wishes to New York's Larry McCarthy, a native of County Cork, who was to become the new President of the GAA. Larry would be the 40th President of the GAA.

Our facilities in February continued to miss the buzz of activity created by training and games. We had missed the special roar of the Rockies since the previous March. We were chomping at the bit to resume normal service. But we had to be patient and keep safe. I encouraged our members to continue to exercise within a 5km radius of home and that before long club activities would resume. I was hoping and praying that before too long I would be engaging with our members and players on the club premises rather than on remote social media outlets.

During the month of February 2021, Austin Stacks was the beneficiary of a generous gesture from Eamonn Linnane Construction. Eamonn, who is a brother-in-law of Éamonn O'Reilly, and a great club supporter, offered to finance an activity in the Club. I explained that I had done the Bracker 100km fundraising walk in July 2020 in order to raise money for a path between the main pitches in Connolly Park, the home of Austin Stacks GAA Club, Tralee. The new path was intended to prevent footfall damage on the pitches and to facilitate all- ability access to the far terrace in Connolly Park. Unfortunately, the amount raised on the walk was not sufficient to cover the cost of the path. Eamonn very kindly agreed to meet with myself and a few of my colleagues in Connolly Park on a Saturday during the month of February so that he could see for himself what I had in mind. Not only did Eamonn agree to lay the path but he also outlined a plan for a path that was far and away more expansive than the one I had in mind. It was indeed a noble gesture and I felt that Austin Stacks was very fortunate to have benefactors like Eamonn Linnane, who were prepared to provide this much needed infrastructure while neither demanding nor expecting anything in return.

CHAPTER TWENTY SIX

DETERIORATING VISION

I was looking forward to my first appointment of 2021 with Mr Flynn on 23rd February. At the time, the coronavirus pandemic was virulent and the HSE was under extreme pressure to cope with the demands being made on it. The February appointment was cancelled and rescheduled for the 13th April 2021. By the time of that appointment, it would have been over four months since I had last visited Mr Flynn and sixteen months since my right cataract had been removed.

During the April appointment, Mr Flynn did a detailed examination of my eyes and felt that I had taken one step forward and one step back. The step forward was the removal of the cataract. The step back was the reduced function in the cornea. The consequences of the step forward and step back was that the vision in my right eye remained unchanged. Mr Flynn said I was in that difficult place where the corrected vision was above the standard necessary to qualify for a driving licence, but the symptoms of the Fuchs Dystrophy were evident and I was becoming more aware of my reducing vision.

We discussed the issue of the corneal transplantation in the right eye as we had done at previous appointments. He told me that he was generally slow to recommend the surgery when the vision meets NDLS driving standard as there are risks with the operation, which means the vision could end up worse over the next few years. I was fully aware of the risks as I had studied the very instructive information that Mr Flynn had given me before Christmas. As Mr Flynn was reassuring about the current standard of my vision, I wasn't particularly pushing for surgery. I had realised much earlier that I wouldn't be making the decision about the time of the next surgery. Mr Flynn was the expert. I knew he would make the decision about operating when he felt it was in my best interests. Because my vision was reasonably functional, Mr Flynn preferred to let some time elapse before he wished to see me again. On my way out, the Practice Co-ordinator slotted me in for an appointment on the 12th October 2021. At the time, that appointment seemed very far away but I knew that I could pick up the phone for an earlier appointment, if I had any concerns.

Mr Flynn also wrote me an updated prescription for eyedrops and suggested that I get distance glasses. However, when I returned to Dr. O'Regan for an eye test, he was of the opinion that distance glasses would not be of any great benefit. I carried on as I had done for some time past. I wore glasses for reading purposes and otherwise, I went without glasses.

During the summer of 2021, I did notice a gradual deterioration in my vision. I always enjoyed reading a daily paper but it was getting progressively more difficult to read small print. I also experienced a lessening of my ability to read text on a television set unless I moved in close to the screen. I was still comfortably reading enlarged print books which I regularly borrowed from my local Library in Tralee but I was now certain that the Fuchs Dystrophy was advancing and the corneas in both my eyes were deteriorating irreversibly.

When the football matches resumed during the summer of 2021, I was shocked by the deterioration in my distance vision. I was scarcely able to read the numbers on the players' jerseys unless they were fairly close to where I was sitting. I positioned myself on the terrace as close to the half-way line as I could get so that I had the best view in both directions. That strategy was helpful for a while but in the autumn of 2021, I was unable to follow the action at either goal mouth or on the far side of the field.

I recall being in the company of some friends at a particular game on our home pitch in Connolly Park. The sun was shining in a cloudless sky and I was having considerable difficulty in reading the scores on our electronic scoreboard. I'm in the habit of keeping a running score in my match programme and doing a tot-up at half time and at full time. On this particular day, I completed my half time accumulated scores but was unable to see if they tallied with the scores on the scoreboard. I turned to one of my companions and inquired of him what the correct score was. I remember his reply, which was made in jest but which resonated with me.

"It's over there on the scoreboard. Are you going blind or what for fucks sake, Mr Chairman?"

I gave him a rueful smile and almost replied that I was going blind for Fuchs sake. I kept my thoughts to myself, however, and excused myself for a bathroom break when I was really moving closer to the scoreboard to see if both scores tallied. That good natured encounter made me realise that to the world at large I looked ship shape and Bristol fashion on the outside but I had a disease that others could not be aware of without I telling them. It made me realise that many other people were also suffering from hidden illnesses but weren't in a hurry to share them with all and sundry. As long as I was able to live a fairly normal life, I wasn't going to make a big deal about my personal situation. I didn't want sympathy or for people to feel they had to look after me in case I might trip-up or suffer some such mishap. I was hoping to have surgery and be restored to good vision before it became public knowledge. The last thing I wanted was for people coming up to me and jokingly remarking that it was a case of the blind leading the blind!

CHAPTER TWENTY SEVEN

GOOD MENTAL HEALTH

In March 2021, Peter Twiss, Secretary, Kerry County Board GAA sent a reminder to all Club Officers, Team Managers, Coaches & Players that the present Covid-19 restrictions, as updated and forwarded by Croke Park to all units of the GAA on 1st Feb 2021, remained in place. The County Secretary stated that all Clubs must ensure that any form of collective training does not take place. Peter also reminded Clubs that all pitches and gyms must remain closed for the time being. Peter added that all GAA people in Kerry were looking forward to the resumption of activities in all Club grounds in the not too-distant-future, but in the meantime, he asked us all to ensure that the health and safety of all within our community was given our full attention.

Austin Stacks had hoped to resume activities in early March. That wouldn't now happen. All our facilities would remain in total lockdown until informed otherwise. As a united club, we had been meticulous in complying with Government and GAA directives to-date and fully supported the sentiments of Peter Twiss. The official position of Austin Stacks GAA Club was that we were in full lockdown and all activities would remain suspended in line with public health and GAA regulations.

Austin Stacks also fully concurred with outgoing GAA President, John Horan's view that the GAA's compliance with public health restrictions was serving the country well. John Horan was justifiably scathing of those who breached training bans and match day protocols, insisting they showed a lack of respect for people's health by their actions. John said that it reflected badly on those who led or allowed those breaches of the regulations to happen. Austin Stacks was very fortunate that no one within our Club would damage its reputation by acting, or by encouraging others to act, in a manner that would breach regulations. So, all of us needed to be patient and to stay safe. We would be restricted to exercising within a 5km radius from home until activities would resume on our own pitches. I felt very sorry for all of our players, especially, and I was very grateful to our entire membership for their exemplary compliance with all the regulations that had, of necessity, been imposed by the Government and the GAA. Deep down, I could hardly wait for an end to this deadly coronavirus pandemic and deeply regretted the havoc been caused by it to the mental health of people throughout the length and breadth of the land.

In the meantime, Éamonn O'Reilly and myself were in the process of finalising a very attractive sponsorship with two well-known local firms, Ned O'Shea & Sons Ltd and John Lane & Sons Ltd. Both firms were very anxious to include a commitment to youth mental health promotion in the package. As this is an issue which was always part of my professional life, I was delighted to do so. Éamonn, who along with being an outstanding Club Vice-Chairman was also the Coaching and Games Development Officer in the club. Good mental health in the coaching and playing cohort was also high-up on his list of priorities.

To get the ball rolling, we organised a virtual one-hour workshop entitled 'One Good Adult' which would be delivered by Jigsaw Kerry, which is a free, non-judgemental, and confidential mental health support service for young people aged 12/25yrs, who are living, working, or studying in County Kerry. Jigsaw Kerry provides guidance and support for young people who are going through a difficult or distressing time. The workshop was scheduled for 8pm on Monday, 19th April 2021.

The aims of the workshop were
(1) To have a greater understanding of mental health and what influences mental health
(2) To recognise the importance of the role of trusted adults in supporting and promoting young people's mental health and
(3) to know how to support and promote the mental health of the young people in their lives.

The workshop was aimed at all senior club players, the parents of all juvenile players, club coaches & club officers and was presented on the

Zoom virtual platform. The timing of the workshop was ideal as mental health was a very topical issue during the lockdown. There was a huge attendance on the night for an outstanding presentation by two superb members of Jigsaw Ireland staff, Caoimhe and Sarah. As Club Chairman, it was a great pleasure for me to introduce a workshop on a topic which was very close to my heart.

I stated that "tonight's Jigsaw Workshop, entitled, One Good Adult, aims to explore the importance of a good adult in the life of a young person. Tonight, we will get an understanding from Caoimhe and Sarah of mental health and the events which determine our quality of mental health. We'll examine the importance of young people having an adult they can trust in their lives. We'll learn how to support and promote youth mental health.

I welcome the association between Jigsaw Kerry and Austin Stacks and I hope that tonight's workshop will be the first of many such events that we share together.

One of the foremost aims of my Executive Committee and myself is to promote positivity and mutual support throughout the club. We support each other and we especially support each and every player who dons the black and amber jersey.

I'd like to thank my colleague, Mike Casey our club's Health and Welfare officer who did a great deal of the organisation for tonight's workshop.

I'd like to sincerely thank Brendan Murphy of Ned O'Shea & Sons Ltd and Pat Lane of John Lane & Sons Ltd who encouraged the link between Jigsaw Kerry and Austin Stacks.

In the near future, Austin Stacks will be formally launching a very generous joint sponsorship by both companies of our U-17, U-15 and U-13 teams. We are very grateful to both companies for this valuable finance, which is exclusively ring fenced for the young players in question. The jerseys worn by the teams in question will carry the slogan JIGSAW KERRY YOUTH MENTAL HEALTH.

I have seen the very impressive design of the new jersey and I'd like to avail of this opportunity to thank my colleague on the Executive Committee, Terry Healy, whose help and expertise with the design was invaluable.

I'll now hand you over to Caoimhe and Sarah for a workshop which you will find very informative and useful in the work that you do with young people. I know that they will both welcome your feedback and comments at the end of their formal presentation."

The workshop was very worthwhile and enjoyable and as Mick Casey said in delivering his words of thanks to the presenters and to all who logged on, this would be the first of the many activities which Austin Stacks would organise to promote positive mental health throughout the club.

CHAPTER TWENTY EIGHT

A NOD & A WINK TO ANTHONY DALY

There was universal welcome in April 2021 for a document issued by Croke Park setting out a general fixtures' framework for an inter-county season commencing in May and concluding at the end of August. For our own Kerry team, the National Football League would begin on the weekend of 15th/16th May, followed by two further rounds in the following fortnight. The league semi-finals would take place on the weekend of 12th/13th June followed by the final on the following weekend. Kerry, Dublin, Galway and Roscommon made up one group.

The Provincial Football Championships would begin on the weekend of 26th/27th June. Munster Championship fixtures were to be issue in the immediate future with the Munster Senior Football Final pencilled in for the weekend of 24th/25th July. The All-Ireland Football Championship semi-finals would take place on the weekend of 14th/15th August and the final would follow on the weekend of 28th/29th August. Austin Stacks was now eagerly awaiting notification from Kerry County Board about the structure and timing of club fixtures. But, at least, the focus was beginning to move from the pandemic to football, hurling and camogie. It was a major step forward on the road to competitions.

Austin Stacks Hurling & Football Club was delighted to host the Meath Senior Hurling team and officials for a training session at Connolly Park at 5pm on Saturday, 22nd May 2021. The Royals were in town to play Kerry in Round Three of the National Hurling League, Division 2A. That game was played at Austin Stack Park, Tralee at 1pm on Sunday, 23rd May.

Austin Stacks was very pleased to welcome the Meath hurlers back to Connolly Park, where the players loosened up for the Kerry game with a puck around, training drills and shooting practice. Austin Stacks had also facilitated the Meath team in 2020, when they weekended in Tralee for a game with Kerry. It was great to see hurling being played on our pitch after an absence of some time.

Our association with the Meath team was part of a concerted effort being made during my term as Chairman, to reactivate hurling in a club which is steeped in hurling tradition dating back to 1928 when Austin Stacks won the Kerry Senior Hurling and Football Championships. Austin Stacks also won the Kerry Senior Hurling Championship in 1929 and another double success in hurling and football was achieved in 1931.

Our senior hurling teams of the late 60's/early 70's, which included the inspirational John Barry, were the unluckiest Rock teams ever, narrowly losing in the county finals of '68, '69 and '74. Our minor hurlers enjoyed county championship success in 1955, 1967 and 1986. Following a series of poor results in the 1990's, our senior team dropped down to the junior ranks, where the club enjoyed considerable success. Austin Stacks hasn't participated in county hurling competitions for a few years.

While our many successes in football from underage to senior, had overshadowed hurling in recent years, I give a firm commitment to do everything in my power during my term as Chairman to rejuvenate Austin Stack's mission to hurling. While the intervention of the coronavirus pandemic had impeded our efforts, the second visit of the Meath team was a big step in the right direction. Now that the Royals had restored the clash of the ash in The Rock, hopefully, it won't be too long before Austin Stacks was back chasing double success in hurling and football.

I had also been very offended by an article written by Anthony Daly, the former Clare hurler, in the Irish Examiner on Monday, 25th May 2020, which suggested that Austin Stacks was not only making no effort to promote hurling in our club but that we were discouraging our players from playing for Tralee Parnells Hurling & Camogie Club. It was a poorly researched article and Mr Daly didn't even do us the courtesy of contact for our point of view before writing the article. I felt very aggrieved for all the fine members of our club who had kept hurling alive in our club for so many years. Éamonn O'Reilly, Tim McMahon and myself felt that Mr Daly's inaccurate comments could not go unanswered so we composed the reply below to vindicate the good name of our club.

"Dear Sir,
An article by Anthony Daly entitled 'Kerry hurling should be helped build their own kingdom' was published in the Irish Examiner on Monday, 25th May 2020. In the course of that article, Mr Daly, for reasons best known to himself, singled out the Austin Stacks GAA Club for unfavourable and inaccurate comment. Austin Stacks, affectionately known as 'The Rock', was founded in 1917 and has ever since, sometimes in very difficult times, worked tirelessly to promote Gaelic football and hurling as well as Irish culture. In its 103 years in existence, The Rock has established a reputation for its high standards, for its exemplary behaviour on and off the field, for its strong community ethos and its successes in both football and hurling.

Today the Austin Stacks GAA Club is in rude health with a very large membership and a dedicate core of administrators and coaches at all level. For over fifty years the club lived a nomadic existence without a permanent home. Thanks to the vision, bravery and foresight of those who preceded us we now have excellent facilities at Connolly Park, Rock St. The Rock has a huge support base, popularly known as 'The Rockies.' Many of our officers, players, mentors, members and supporters have deep roots in The Rock. Many new families have become valued members of our club because of its reputation for excellence and the duty of care it exercises for its entire membership.

In his article, Mr Daly claims to have 'heard a story recently that didn't surprise me in the least. The best U-12 hurler in Kerry is a highly talented dual player from Tralee, who hurls with Parnells and kicks football with Austin Stacks. Stacks got such a panic attack that the young lad may become distracted by hurling that they got one of their highly-respected former Kerry footballers to have a word in his year. How paranoid would you have to be to try and turn a 12year old?'

We would humbly suggest that Anthony Daly is the person suffering from paranoia if he believes a tall-tale like that from an anonymous source. That is not the Rock way. Sport is the antidote to antisocial behaviour and we fully support the campaign for sport, recreation and leisure. Naturally, we hope that football will be the first sport of choice for all our players but we are well aware that the majority of our players enjoy other sports. And so, it should be. Tralee is a mecca of sports to suit all tastes – football, hurling, camogie, handball, basketball, golf, cricket, athletics, cycling, swimming, squash, to mention just a few. All of the sports clubs in Tralee and Kerry do good work. Indeed, if our 'highly-respected former Kerry footballer' had to have a word in the ear of every Austin Stacks player who played other sports, he'd be out and about from first light until the stars come out!

The Rock is particularly proud of its juvenile section, the jewel in the crown of a great club. Mr Daly posed the question 'should Stacks not be more worried about trying to recruit young lads ahead of O'Rahillys, Mitchels and Na Gaeil - the other clubs in the town – instead of telling one of their own to turn his back on hurling and his friends?' Not at all, we are happy with our fair share and, as mentioned above, hurling is part of the Rock DNA. All of the GAA clubs in Tralee coexist in a spirit of mutual respect and cooperation. The clubs are rivals on the field of play but there are longstanding acquaintances and friendships off the field. We are all motivate by the same desire to promote the aims and values of the GAA. The majority of our academy intake comes from Rock families. We also hold an annual registration and parents evening where all families are welcome to enrol their children. The vast majority of youngsters – boys and girls – remain loyal to Austin Stacks throughout their entire lives.

While our Senior men's and ladies' club as well as our Juvenile Club are thriving, in recent years there has been a regrettable decline in our hurling section. Our hurling teams were very competitive since our foundation and Austin Stacks was in effect a Tralee and local area hurling team. Players from our neighbouring clubs donned the black and amber to play hurling with the Rock. We were privileged to have them on our teams and they united the entire town of Tralee and further afield behind our hurling teams. People like Kerry football star, Niall Sheehy of John Mitchels, Rugby International Dick Spring of Kerins O Rahillys and the late Joe O Sullivan of West Kerry, to mention but a few, have done The Rock some service on the hurling field. While Austin Stacks has not had the numbers to compete in hurling competitions for a few years, we are pleased to support the initiative of the new Tralee Parnells Hurling and Camogie Club in promoting those games in the Tralee area. That club is now effectively doing what Austin Stacks did for many years. We are delighted that any of our players, who are interested in hurling, now have a local hurling club on their doorstep. Likewise, Austin Stacks, has always accommodated players from hurling only clubs, who wish to play football with our club.

To the best of our knowledge, Anthony Daly has never set foot in Connolly Park. He has never seen how our wonderful club goes about its business. He wrote a very poorly researched article based on a nod and a wink. He did Austin Stacks a grave injustice. If he'd like to soak up the exhilarating atmosphere in Connolly Park and meet with the 'rare auld stock of the Rock,' he'd be more than welcome to visit Austin Stacks at any time."

The response was signed by myself as Chairman of Austin Stacks GAA Club, Éamonn O Reilly, Vice- Chairman, Austin Stacks GAA Club and Tim McMahon, Chairman, Austin Stacks Juvenile GAA Club. Needless to say, Anthony Daly never took up our invitation to visit our vibrant club. Neither did he name the anonymous person who fed him false information nor the highly-respected former Kerry footballer who was reputedly sent out to discourage a highly talented youngster from playing with Parnells. Every mother's son knew the identity of the Kerry and Austin Stacks football star referred to by Mr Daly. You'd have to travel a long way to find a man with more integrity, openness and honesty. That highly-respected former Kerry footballer was done a great injustice in Anthony Daly's article. It reminded me of the old Irish adage about gossip – 'dúirt bean liom go ndúirt bean léi!' – which translates as 'a woman told me that a woman told her!'

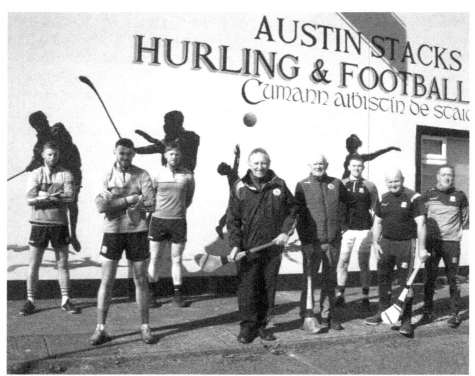

Billy Ryle, Club Chairman and Jim Naughton, Chairman Field Committee, centre, welcomed the Meath Hurling team for a puck around on Saturday, 22nd May 2021 prior to their national hurling league fixture with Kerry on the following day

CHAPTER TWENTY NINE

ONE GOOD ADULT TO LISTEN

One of the very special memories, I have about my time as Chairman of Austin Stacks, was the official launch on Sunday, 30th May 2021 of a new three-year sponsorship of our under-age teams in glorious sunshine at Connolly Park. In my address, I said that I was delighted to announce that Ned O'Shea & Sons Construction Ltd and John Lane & Sons Ltd, Food Service Distributors, would jointly sponsor Austin Stacks U-17, U-15 and U-13 football teams – six teams in total – for a three-year period beginning this current year. Both companies were providing a financial package for teams and related expenditure.

I added that it was a pleasure for Austin Stacks to be associated with two long established Kerry based companies in promoting the club's aims and objectives. I thanked both companies for providing Austin Stacks with the financial support to maintain and improve the service that the club provides for its young players. I especially thanked Benny Murphy of Ned O'Shea & Sons Construction Ltd and Pat Lane of John Lane & Sons Ltd, Food Service Distributors who were a pleasure to negotiate with from the outset.

I welcomed the partnership with Jigsaw Kerry. "In these very stressful times for young people, nothing could be more appropriate" I said. "Austin Stacks has established a formal working relationship with Jigsaw Kerry, which is a free, non-judgemental and confidential mental health support service for young people aged 12-25 years living, working or studying in Co. Kerry. The jerseys of the six sponsored teams will display the logo, 'Jigsaw Kerry Youth Mental Health' and Austin Stacks is also availing of the expertise of Jigsaw Kerry to provide mental health information, support and counselling for team members, both individually and in groups."

Benny Murphy replying on behalf of joint-sponsors, Ned O Shea & Sons Ltd and John Lane & Sons Ltd stated that both companies were delighted to provide a financial package to Austin Stacks at a time when it was difficult to fund under age activities. The sponsorship would help to pay for the new jerseys as well as essential equipment. The sponsors were keen also, Benny added, that the funding would also enable the young players to enjoy a few social days out where friendships could develop and team bonding could take place.

Neither company was too interested in self-promotion nor in having their logos dominating the new jerseys, Benny said. Instead, they were using the sponsorship to promote the wonderful work of Jigsaw Kerry, which provides a fantastic range of supports for young people with issues of mental health. Both companies were very pleased to have the Jigsaw Kerry logo on the front of the jerseys. That exposure would create awareness of the availability of the service to those who may need support in dealing with the various issues that young people encounter.

Frank O Rahilly of Jigsaw Kerry said he was delighted to be present at the launch. He referenced the many successes which Austin Stacks had enjoyed on the field. He added that he had great admiration for the club and the standards under which it operates. "Austin Stacks was now adding a new dimension to a GAA club by extending player welfare to activities off the field. Jigsaw Kerry was thrilled," Frank said "to be promoting positive mental health in a great club. Jigsaw Kerry emphasises early intervention and prevention when dealing with youth mental health. He said no problem was too small. It may be a major concern for the young person who has it. Austin Stacks coaches are promoting positive mental health every time they work with the young players. The coaches can see exactly where young people are and what needs they have."

Frank said that the best method of reaching out to a young person is to listen actively to what the young person is saying. Each young person needs one good adult in her/his life who makes time available to be a listener. Jigsaw Kerry would now work with Austin Stacks in promoting positive mental health through workshops, team talks and individual counselling. Frank said that Jigsaw Kerry was delighted to be a partner with the sponsors and Austin Stacks in this very progressive initiative. "Mol an óige agus tiocfaidh sé," he concluded.

Éamonn O'Reilly and myself had worked very hard to secure that juvenile sponsorship. It meant that the Juvenile Club now had adequate funding for the comprehensive program it provided for young people year after year. As a Career and Educational Counsellor, I was overjoyed by the link with Jigsaw Kerry. I was very impressed also by Frank O Rahilly. From our first meeting, Frank struck me as a man who was determined to provide a first-rate mental health service to the young people of Kerry. I had no doubt that Frank's association with Austin Stacks through this sponsorship would be of tremendous benefit to our young players.

The jerseys of the six sponsored teams were now displaying the logo, Jigsaw Kerry Youth Mental Health. Because of the outstanding working relationship which has been established by Mike Casey, our Health & Safety Officer, with Jigsaw Kerry our young people are availing of mental health information, support and counselling when required. This sponsorship offered Austin Stacks a great deal more than money. Benny Murphy and Pat Lane brought a new dimension to team sponsorship.

There was further good new towards the end of May 2021 when the general fixtures were released for our Senior A, B and C teams. Our Senior A team would have five games in Division 1A of the season's curtailed County League - three home games against Dingle (w/e 12th/13th June), John Mitchels (w/e 17th/18th July) and Kilcummin (w/e 31st July/1st August) and two away games against Spa (w/e 19th/20th June) and Dr. Crokes (w/e 3rd/4th July). The County Senior League Division One final would be between the top teams in Division 1A and Division 1B. An Ghaeltacht, Beaufort, Kenmare Shamrocks, Kerins O'Rahillys, Killarney Legion and Rathmore were drawn in Division 1B. I was very happy with the draw and was very confident that we could retain that title in a bid for a clean sweep of the three senior titles in County Kerry.

Our Senior B team which was playing in Division Five A of the County League would be at home against Moyvane and Ballyduff and away to Laune Rangers, Kilgarven and Foilmore. I was very keen for this team to do well in their league. The had an excellent management team in Paddy Barry (Manager), Éamonn O Reilly, Kieran Kelliher, Mikey Collins, Tim Mc Mahon, TJ Sheehan and Dale Counihan. The winners of Division Five A and Five B would be promoted. I dearly wanted this team to achieve promotion to Division Four and to win the Division Five final.

Austin Stacks had also entered our Senior B and Senior C teams in the 2021 leagues in the amalgamated St. Brendan's District Board and the Tralee District Board. I was delighted with this new competition as it would provide games for our Senior C team in what was likely to be a curtailed season. Our Senior C squad, popularly known as Charlie's Angels, is full of energy and excitement and is a healthy blend of up-and-coming young footballers and of those who still enjoy playing at a more leisurely level. Their team manager is the charismatic Aidan O'Connor, former Club Chairman and recently elected Club President at the AGM on the 15th January 2023. Group A contained Ardfert B, Austin Stacks B, Kerins O'Rahilly's B & John Mitchel's B. Drawn in Group B were Austin Stacks C, Ballymac B, Churchill B and St. Pat's B. The competition would begin on Tuesday, 22nd June 2021 with further games on the 29th June and the 6th July.

It was wonderful to see our teams back on the field training, albeit under strict regulations. It wouldn't be long before the games got under way for players at all levels. I could hardly wait as I had a very good feeling about what lay ahead.

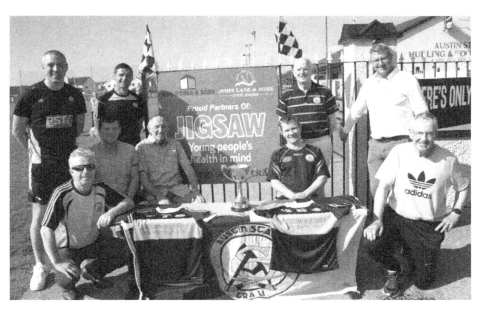

At the launch of the Austin Stack Juvenile Club joint sponsorship by Ned O Shea & Co Ltd and John Lane & Co Ltd on the 30th May 2021 were Front L/r: Éamonn O Reilly, (Vice-Chairman), Frank O'Rahilly (Jigsaw Kerry), Billy Ryle (Chairman), Tim McMahon (Juvenile Chairman) and Colm Mangan (Club Executive Committee). Back L/r Kieran Donaghy (Senior Player), Wayne Quillinan (Senior Team Manager), Jim Naughton (Chairman, Field Committee) and Benny Murphy (Ned O Shea & Co)

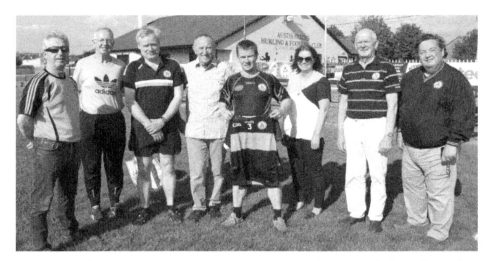

Austin Stacks Executive Committee members who attended the launch of the Juvenile Club joint sponsorship by Ned O Shea & Co Ltd and John Lane & Co Ltd on the 30th May 2021. L/r Éamonn O'Reilly, Colm Mangan, Shane Lynch, Billy Ryle, Tim McMahon, Mary Fitzmaurice, Jim Naughton and Eddie Barrett

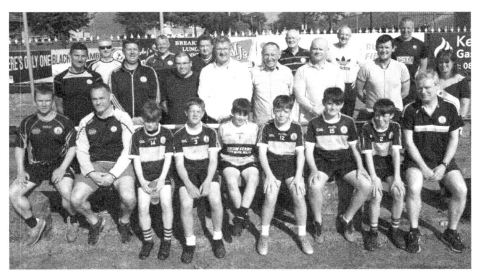

Group photo taken with Benny Murphy (4th left second row) and Pat Lane (6th left second row) at the launch of the Austin Stack Juvenile Club joint sponsorship by Ned O Shea & Co Ltd and John Lane & Co Ltd on the 30th May 2021

Front from left: Tim McMahon, Pa Laide, David Hobbert, Rian Walsh, Eoghan Murphy, Rory Lynch, Barry Laide, Darragh Lyons & Shane Lynch

Middle from left: Wayne Quillinan, Joe Walsh, Ger Hobbert, Benny Murphy, Billy Ryle, Pat Lane, Frank O Rahilly & Mary Fitzmaurice

Back from left: Éamonn O Reilly, Ciarán Murphy, Eddie Barrett, Jim Naughton, Colm Mangan & Kieran Donaghy

CHAPTER THIRTY

DISABILITY PATH

With the summer fast approaching Austin Stacks relaunched its JobMatch program. JobMatch was devised by a small committee consisting of then Club Chairman, Liam Lynch, Éamonn O'Reilly, Catherine Ryan and myself some years earlier to support our members in securing employment locally by liaising with local employers who might have job opportunities available. JobMatch catered for our home-based members and it also provided job opportunities for members, who were working elsewhere in Ireland or abroad and who were anxious to relocate home. We reached out each year to the local business community for details of any jobs that they had available. Each year, we identified some fantastic opportunities around short-term summer work and permanent employment. These jobs ranged across the services, tourism, retail, industrial and professional sectors. We regular sourced employment opportunities for members who had recently completed their second or third level education and who were in search of employment locally. We also facilitated members who were looking for a change of career or a return to the region. We began by inviting any member who was seeking employment to submit a Curriculum Vitae. We then matched the skills set of the job seeker to the employment positions that were available. My primary function on the JobMatch committee was to assist members in building well prepared CV's, to identify their career and personal skills and to prioritise their preferred types of employment. I also prepared them for interview and put each job seeker through a formal practice interview before meeting any potential employer. As a professional Career Guidance Counsellor, I also provided confidential counselling to any member who raised issue of concern during our one-on-one sessions. I found my role on the JobMatch committee to be very satisfying. I was assisting our members to find good quality employment. I helped them to resolve issues of a personal nature which were causing them some concern or distress. Of course, JobMatch was primarily focussed on keeping our players at home or bringing home those who were anxious to return. JobMatch is still providing a great service to Austin Stacks members and Mike Casey, Siobhán Power and George Dineen have been invaluable additions to the committee.

I felt very proud when our new disability path was blessed and officially opened on a beautiful evening on the 17th July, 2021 before our vital Senior County League Division One game against local rivals, John Mitchels. Just a year before on the 17th July, 2020, I had begun the 10-day Bracker 100km fundraising walk on the Bracker O'Regan Road. The purpose of the walk was to raise funds for a path allowing access to the far side of the main pitch and to reduce footfall on the pitches. I was very grateful to those who had helped me to organise the walk, to those who walked with me and to those who had contributed so generously.

In my words of welcome at the opening I said that I was very grateful to Eamonn Linnane Construction and his team for building the beautiful path which facilitated access to the far terrace in Connolly Park for people of all abilities. My fundraising walk had come up short of the amount needed to lay the path but Eamonn had very kindly offered to do the work cost free. It was an altruistic gesture from a man who wanted no thanks but, who certainly deserved thanks on the night. I added that all Rock supporters could now be part of the 16th Man on the Árd Carraig Terrace.

"My sincere thanks to Fr. Amos Ruto for joining us to bless the path and all present. I assure you, Father, that most of us are badly in need of your blessing! When Fr Amos first came to town, he was based at St John's Presbytery, at the John Mitchels' side of town. No doubt, he was fed a lot of tall tales about their brilliant footballers and their famous five in a row Kerry Senior Football Championship winning team. Fortunately, Fr Pádraig Walsh, our local Parish priest, rescued him and settled him into St. Brendan's Presbytery at the top of the Rock, the Street of Champions, the home of pure football. So, I hope that Fr Amos is by now a true Rockie and backing the Stacks against the Mitchels in tonight's game," I added.

Proving that life is full of bitter-sweet occasions I referred to a recent sad occurrence. "Also, in our blessing this evening, I'd like Fr. Amos to include a proud and dedicated colleague, the great Jo Jo Barrett, who died earlier today. May he rest in peace."

"Nobody could be more appropriate to cut the ribbon than George Dineen, a lifelong Rockie supporter and a valued member of our Club community. While his disability didn't allow him to play football, he was always a member of the team. I was shown a lovely picture during the week of George and his friends celebrating an underage success and George was the proudest man in the picture. George is ever present at Stacks games and his positive outlook and zest for live are infectious. George represents all that is good about Austin Stacks and he inspires us to make Connolly Park as accessible as possible to our members of all abilities." I concluded.

Fr Amos then blessed the path and all of us in attendance. He also showed that he had already acquired some of the legendary Irish roguery by saying,

"Tonight, I will be neutral in the match because I have many good friends in both clubs."

George then cut the ribbon to formally open the path. Who else could be the first man to cross the path other than George, who was pushed along the fabulous new path in his wheelchair by his dad, also called George and a former Chairman of Austin Stacks. The new path was one of my finest achievements during my term as Chairman of Austin Stacks.

When that pleasant ceremony had concluded it was my duty as Club Chairman to turn to a task which would be emotional but a rare honour for me. Jo Jo Barrett, a man who epitomised all that was good about Austin Stacks, had passed to his eternal reward earlier in the day. My oration before the game was an inadequate attempt to capture the career of a very special man.

"Even though he had been ill for some time, it was with shock and sadness that we learned this morning of the passing of our friend and colleague, Jo Jo Barrett, one of Austin Stacks greatest clubmen.

Jo Jo's family is steeped in Rock history. His late father Joe, his uncles, Tommy, John and Eddie and his brothers Tim and John all played with Austin Stacks and Kerry. His uncle Christy was one of the founding members of the Rock Club in 1917. Jo Jo's son, Joe also played with the Rock in the early nineties.

Jo Jo made his Senior County Championship debut with Austin Stacks at the tender age of sixteen years on the 7th June 1959. He played for seventeen consecutive seasons, winning Senior County Championship medals in 1973 and 1976. During Jo Jo's early playing days, the Rock was going through a barren period but with players like Jo Jo on the scene to inspire the younger players coming up through the ranks, prospects of success were getting better and better. There was no prouder man in Austin Stack Park on that October Sunday in 1973 when Austin Stacks bridged a 37-year gap to win its sixth Senior Football Championship title.

Like his father before him, Jo Jo also donned the Kerry jersey, winning an All-Ireland Senior Football medal in 1962 and an under-21 medal in 1964. Jo Jo was a member of the Kerry Senior Football panel from 1962 to 1965. He made his debut when coming on as a substitute in the 1962 All-Ireland final against Roscommon. He won four Munster Championship Senior Football medals during that period and he lined out at left full forward in the 1964 and 1965 All-Ireland Senior Football Championships against Galway.

When his playing days were ended, Jo Jo managed Austin Stacks Senior Football team for two seasons, culminating in the club's most historic win to-date, the 1977 All-Ireland Senior Club Championship Final. He also served as Club Chairman in 1977 and 1978. Later, after he had moved to Dublin as a Sports Journalist with the Evening Herald, he managed a number of teams, including the Wexford Senior Football team.

In 1977, he wrote a masterpiece of a book, entitled 'In the name of the game' inspired by a conversation which he had. as a nine-year-old boy, with his dying father in 1952. The book outlines how hurling and football played a major role in reuniting players who found themselves on different sides during the Civil War of 1922/23 and how they remained life-long friends thereafter, players like his own father, Joe, and Con Brosnan of Moyvane.

On behalf of the entire membership of Austin Stacks and on my own behalf, I extend sincere sympathy to Jo Jo's family and friends.

Slán leat, Jo Jo, a chara agus ar dhéis lámh Dé go raibh d'anam dílis.

Please join me in observing a minute's silence as a matter of respect for an outstanding Austin Stacks and Kerry stalwart."

In the game that followed Austin Stacks defeated John Mitchels by 0-14 to 0-11 to end a day of mixed emotions for me. On Sunday afternoon, I visited Jo Jo's family and spent some time with his remains at the home of his daughter, Noelle in Barrow, Ardfert. Because of the HSE guidelines in operation at the time, Austin Stacks provided a standing guard of honour at Mulchinock's Corner, Upper Rock St as Jo Jo's funeral cortége made its way to Clogher Cemetery.

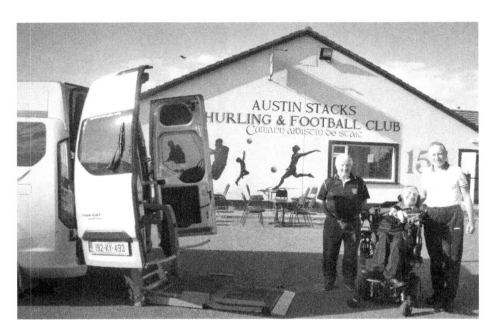

Austin Stacks Club Chairman, Billy Ryle, right, welcomes guest of honour, George Dineen and his dad, George to the official opening of the new all-abilities path at the Club's Connolly Park Grounds on the 17th July 2021

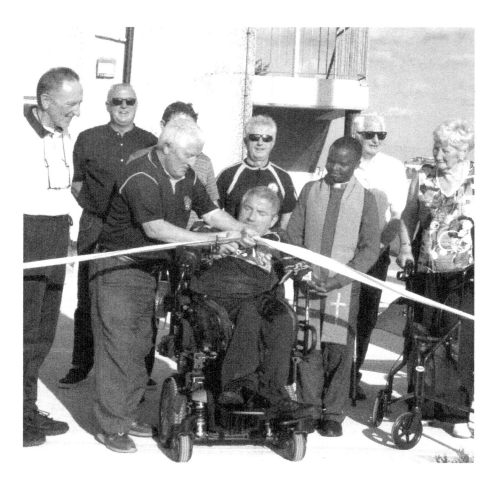

George Dineen, seated, cuts the ribbon to officially open the all-abilities path at the Austin Stacks Club Grounds on the 17th July 2021. Pictured behind from left are Billy Ryle (Club Chairman), John Tobin, George Dineen Snr, Éamonn Linnane (Sponsor), Éamonn O'Reilly (Club Vice-Chairman), Fr Amos Roto, Denis O'Regan and Mairéad Fernane

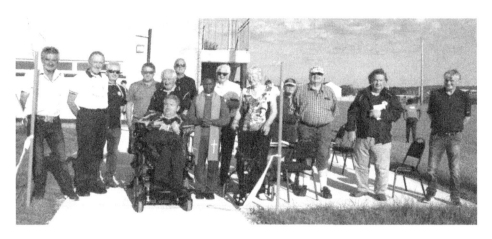

At the official opening of the new all-abilities path at the Austin Stacks Club Grounds on the 17th July 2021were, in front, Guest of Honour, George Dineen who cut the ribbon. Back L/r: John Breen, Billy Ryle, Éamonn O'Reilly, Éamonn Linnane, George Dineen Snr, John Tobin, Fr Amos Roto, who blessed the new path, Denis O'Regan, Mairéad Fernane, Martin Collins, Tim Guiheen, Eddie Barrett and Noel O'Connell

CHAPTER THIRTY ONE

PROMOTION FOR SENIOR B TEAM

By mid-July the club was fully engaged with football competitions and as we were approaching the business end of the season, I requested every member and supporter of Austin Stacks to give total backing to our teams and mentors in their quest for success on the field of play. It was due time to show the rock-solid support for our teams for which Austin Stacks supporters are famous. Positive vocal encouragement from the 16th man on the terraces would let the players and mentors know that the Rockies were fully behind them. It was one for all and all for one in our determination to bring success to the club. I appealed to our supporters to let the players know that their efforts were appreciated. I asked them to let the players know that an off-target scoring attempt or a missed tackle wouldn't be faulted. I asked them to remember that every player who dons the black & amber jersey gives his all for the team. Every mentor wants his team to win. Every supporter could help the effort by not criticising players or mentors during the course of a game. By standing shoulder to shoulder with our teams and mentors, we would add more titles to those that were so hard-won the previous year.

I must admit that the early season form of our senior team was beginning to worry me. We secured a hard-earned point on the 12th June 2021 at home against Dingle in our first outing in the County Senior League, Division One. In a low scoring game, we scored 0-9 to 1-6 for Dingle. The following week, on the 19th June we travelled to play Spa, Killarney. Despite leading by 1-10 to 0-1 as we approached halftime, we had to depend on a last-minute equaliser to leave for home with a single point. The final score was Austin Stacks 1-13 Spa 2-10. We returned to Killarney on the 3rd July where we lost to Dr Crokes on a score of ten points for the home side against our nine points. As mentioned early, we got a home win against John Mitchels on the 17th July. I thought we played our best league game on home soil on the 1st August when we beat Kilcummin on a scoreline of 1-13 to 1-11.

After playing all five rounds of the Senior County League, Division One, Austin Stacks had chalked up six points out of a possible ten. That points total wasn't good enough to put us on top of the table in Group A. We were eliminated from the County Senior League and my hopes of winning all three senior titles in 2021 were dashed.

Our Senior B team, on the other hand was in blistering form in Division Five of the County League. The team got off to a flying start by winning away to Laune Rangers by a whopping 6-10 to 1-7 on the 13th June 2021. A week later on the 20th June the team had a hard-fought home win against Moyvane by 2-11 to 3-6. On the following Tuesday evening, 22nd June, the team had a convincing win away to Kerins O'Rahillys in the Tralee and St Brendan's Districts league on a scoreline of 4-7 to 1-9.

It was back to County League duty in Kilgarvan on the 4th July where Austin Stacks scored 1-12 to the home side's 0-8. Ballyduff arrived, unbeaten after three games, to Connolly Park on the 18th July. In a tough encounter our team dug very deep to win by 1-11 to 0-9. Two days later, on the 20th July, our unbeaten Senior B team won the club's first trophy of the season when they captured the inaugural Tralee and St. Brendan's League title by defeating Kerins O'Rahillys, our visitors to Connolly Park, by 0-10 points to 0-5. It was now all to play for in our final County League game away against St Michael's Foilmore on Saturday evening, 31st July. A win would see our team promoted to Division Four as well as qualifying the team for the League Final against Cordal, the winners of the other group. It was a tough ask but this team didn't know how to lose and I looked forward to a trip to South Kerry.

As my eye sight was continuing to deteriorate, my wife, Sheila drove me down to Foilmore on a beautiful Saturday evening on 31st July for our 7pm game against the home side, St. Michael's. The home support was out in force while our travelling support mainly consisted of parents and friends of our players. I accepted that this game didn't have the same appeal as a Division One game, but as promotion to Division Four was at stake, I would have appreciated the presence of a greater number of Austin Stacks supporters. At least, the dug-outs were on the far side of the pitch from the Stand and that worked to the advantage of our players and mentors. I sat in an almost empty Stand with Canice and Deirdre Walsh, whose son Shane played a blinder on the night.

This game turned out to be our toughest test to-date. Austin Stacks were behind by five points to one at the first water break. But whatever Paddy Barry and his colleagues put in the water during that first break certainly worked the oracle as we scored four points to two for St Michaels during the second quarter. The score was 0-7 to 0-5 in favour of the home side at half-time. By the end of the third quarter the teams were level at 0-8 each. It was all to play for in the final quarter.

The teams were still level at 0-9 each with six minutes remaining. It was heart stopping stuff as each side chased the win. The game dramatically changed in our favour when Gearóid Fitzgerald hit the back of the net for a lead that was never going to be surrendered. After a heroic effort Austin Stacks won the game and promotion to Division Four by 1-10 to 0-10.

There was joy unconfined as we celebrated together on the field after the game. The Senior B team just kept giving and giving. We would ask them to give one more time against Cordal in the Division Five League Final. This game was initially fixed for Farranfore on Saturday, 7th August at 7pm but was rescheduled for Sunday, 22nd August. I felt that a game of this stature should be played at a venue with good facilities for teams and supporters and I made a request to Kerry County Board to play the game in Castleisland, which was convenient for both teams. My request was granted and, as I had hoped, Austin Stacks supporters travelled in large numbers to Castleisland on a pleasant Sunday evening.

The game was a tough uncompromising one between two evenly matched teams. We started well and led by 0-7 to 0-3 after the first quarter. Cordal dominated the second quarter to lead at halftime by 0-9 to 0-8. At the end of the third quarter, it was 0-13 to 0-12 in favour of Cordal. But as they had done all season, our gallant team members delivered one more time by outscoring the opposition by 2-4 to 1-0 in the final quarter. Austin Stacks Senior B team were Senior County League, Division Five champions on a final score of 2-16 to 1-13 and were on their way to Division Four.

There was a huge cheer when the winning trophy was presented to team captain, Rory Forbes by Liam Lynch, County Board Development Officer. The 'Man of the Match' award went deservedly to our centre-back, Paul Galvin. This wonderful squad of players had delivered two prestigious titles to our club. They had done their club proud. I was also very grateful to the team's mentors Paddy Barry (Manager), Éamonn O'Reilly, Kieran Kelliher Tim McMahon, Dale Counihan, Mikey Collins and TJ Sheehan and. It was now time to focus on another double, the Senior Club Championship and the County Senior Football Championship.

On Wednesday, 1st September 2021, I sat down with senior team Manager, Wayne Quillinan and Coach and Games Development Manager, Éamonn O'Reilly, who was also Club Vice Chairman, for a review of the season and a frank and honest exchange of views. Each of us spoke openly and cordially and by meetings end we all sang from the hymn sheet of senior team success in the two upcoming competitions. With games coming fast and furious during the Senior Club Championship and the County Senior Championship following fast on the heels of that competition, the Divisional sides would be vulnerable. This was the year for a club side to become County Senior Football Champions. I was determined that that club side would be Austin Stacks.

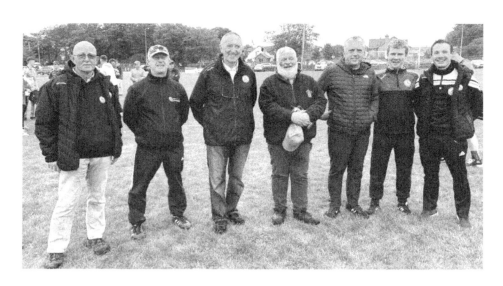

Austin Stacks Club Chairman Billy Ryle, third from left, pictured with the Senior B management team, which won the Senior County League Division Five Final by defeating Cordal in Castleisland on the 22nd August 2021. L/r TJ Sheehan, Éamonn O'Reilly, Billy Ryle, Paddy Barry, Kieran Kelliher, Tim McMahon and Mikey Collins

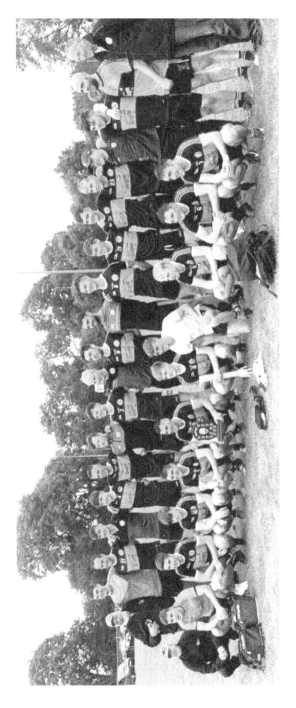

Austin Stacks Senior B team which won the Senior County League Division Five Final by defeating Cordal in Castleisland on the 22nd August 2021
Front L/r Éamonn O'Reilly, Club Vice-Chairman, Calvin Foley, Conor Myres, Cian Purcell, Luke Chester, Rory Forbes, Evan Foley, Seán Ryan, Gearóid Sheehan, Paul Galvin and Andrew Morrissey
Back L/r Paddy Barry, Team Manager, Ben Quilter, Paul Barrett, Dean Rusk, Rory O'Connell, Niall Fitzmaurice, Ciarán O'Connell, Shane Walsh, Joey Nagle, Dara Barry Walsh, Gearóid Fitzgerald, Eoghan Carroll, Tom O'Farrell, Greg Scanlon, Dean Scanlan, Adam Curran, Dan O'Rourke, David Hennessy and Billy Ryle, Club Chairman

CHAPTER THIRTY TWO

THREE IN A ROW SENIOR CLUB CHAMPIONS

Austin Stacks was drawn in Group A of the 2021 Senior Club Championship along with Dingle, Kerins O'Rahillys and Killarney Legion. Group B comprised Dr. Crokes, Kenmare Shamrocks, Templenoe and the 2020 Intermediate Football Championship winners, who were as yet unknown. Each team would have three games, one each at a neutral venue, a home venue and an away venue. Our neutral venue game was to be in Round One against Legion, Killarney. Each winner of round one games would be at home for the second game and away for the third game. The winners of each group would have home advantage in the semi-finals and play the runners-up in the opposite group. The final would then take place at a neutral venue. That meant it would take five games for Austin Stacks to win that competition for the third consecutive year. I was confident that we could do so.

Austin Stacks started very impressively in our first game in the Senior Club Championship against the Legion which was played in Castleisland on Sunday, 5th September. 2021. With Joe O Connor prominent in his first outing after his league campaign with Kerry, The Rock led at halftime by 0-8 to 0-3. Legion succeeded in scoring only five points in the second half, while we tagged on 1-6, which include a super goal from Brendan O Sullivan. Final score was Austin Stacks 1-14 Legion 0-8.

On Sunday, 12th September we hosted Kerins O'Rahillys in Connolly Park in what can only be described as a typical derby clash where no quarter was given and where none was asked for. We just shaded the first half by 0-6 to 0-5 but at the end of the third quarter O'Rahillys held a two-point advantage, 0-10 to 0-8 after a dominant spell. But Austin Stacks produced its best form in the final quarter to win the game by 1-13 to 0-12. Second half substitute Darragh O'Brien made the difference by scoring three points and also finding the net from the penalty spot.

We travelled to Dingle on Sunday, 26th September, 2021 in the knowledge that both teams were already through to the semi-finals of the senior club championship. There was still a lot to play for, as the team that won this match would have home venue in the semi-final. As well as that, Dingle had won the County Senior League, Division One title earlier in the year, so victory in Dingle would give our team a huge confidence boost. For most of the game it looked as if the win was beyond us. After an indifferent first half we trailed by 0-4 to 1-8. Thing didn't look much brighter after 10 minutes of the second half when Dingle led by 2-9 to 1-4. Just as we were beginning to despair, the Austin Stacks team was transformed and produced a superb final twenty minutes to win by 2-12 to 2-10.

Our semi-final against Templenoe, which was played on a beautiful autumnal afternoon in Connolly Park on Sunday, 10th October, 2021 was a total anti-climax. A low-scoring first half was close enough with our team shading it by 0-4 to 0-2. The second half was very one-sided with Templenoe scoring just another two points compared to our impressive 3-5. A tougher game might have been a better preparation for the final but, as the saying goes, you can only play the team that's facing you. Final score was 3-9 to 0-4. We had qualified for our third consecutive senior club final. The game was fixed for Fitzgerald Stadium, Killarney on Sunday, 17th October 2021. Our opponents would be Kenmare Shamrocks, the team we had beaten in the 2020 final at the same venue.

Two days after our game with Templenoe, on the 12th October 2021, I returned to Cork for my first appointment with Mr Flynn since I had last visited the Elysian on the 13th April 2021. My vision had considerable deteriorated and I was struggling to follow the action on the football field. But more about that in the next Chapter.

Austin Stacks supporters flocked to Killarney on Sunday, 17th October 2021 to support their team in the senior club final. The Rockies are famous for the colour and razzamatazz they display on the terrace. Austin Stack values it's supporters whose vocal and drum support provides plenty of encouragement to our teams during games. I was very pleased to see them in their customary position on the far terrace in Killarney. They paraded into the stadium to the sound of drums and confidently marched along the terrace across from the stand. They looked intimidating and I was very glad that they were our supporters.

The experts tell us that goals win matches and we were lucky enough to score an early goal which gave us a lead which we never relinquished. We were ahead by 1-3 to 0-4 at the first water-break. After an equally contested second quarter where each side added on three points each, we retained our two points lead, 1-6 to 0-7. Austin Stacks was the dominant team in the third quarter where we scored four points to two for Kenmare. We now led by 1-10 to 0-9 with just the final quarter to be played. We quickly increased our lead to six points on the resumption of play but Kenmare replied immediately with a goal to half our lead, 1-12 to 1-9. Our team kept its composure, however and we ran out as deserving winners over a gallant Kenmare Shamrocks team on a final scoreline of 1-16 to 1-11. It was wonderful to watch Captain Fantastic, Dylan Casey receiving the cup from Kerry County Board Chairman, Tim Murphy. Our Kerry star, Joe O'Connor, who played a blinder, was a worthy recipient of the 'Man of The Match' award. Our own club 'Man of The Match' award went to Jack O' Shea, who was displaying the best form of his life.

I was very proud of our Senior A squad for winning their third consecutive senior club title. Now it was time to focus on the blue riband competition, Kerry Senior Football Championship. The common consensus was that Austin Stacks was the best club team in Kerry, but that the County Championship was the preserve of the big Divisional sides like Mid-Kerry, St. Brendan's, South Kerry and especially East Kerry, who had the brilliant Clifford brothers in their ranks and looked unbeatable on paper. East Kerry had the pick of nine or ten clubs in their divisional area and many of their squad had inter-county experience.

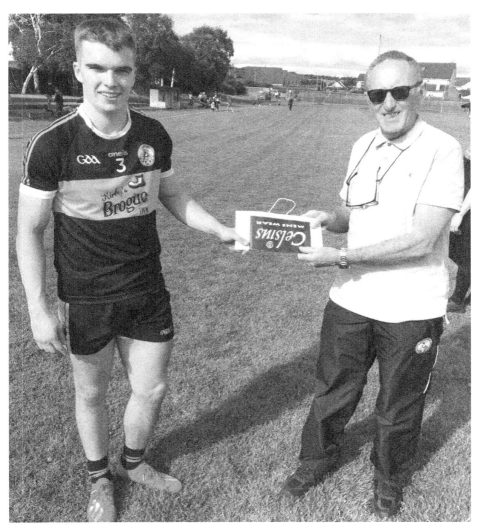

Billy Ryle, Austin Stacks Club Chairman, presents the Celsius Menswear 'Man of the Match' award to Dylan Casey after Austin Stacks win over Kerins O'Rahillys on 12th September 2021

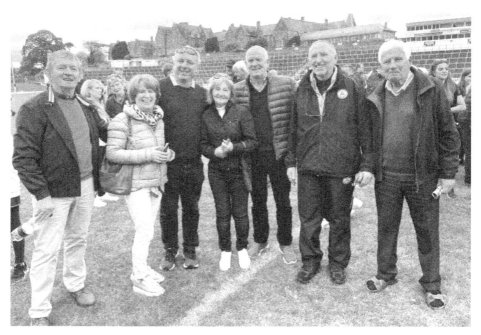

A happy group of Austin Stacks supporters pictured in Killarney on the 17th October 2021 after the victory over Kenmare Shamrocks in the Kerry Senior Club Final. L/r Nial & Maura Shanahan, Ed O Brien, Joan & Jim Naughton, Billy Ryle and Pat Murphy

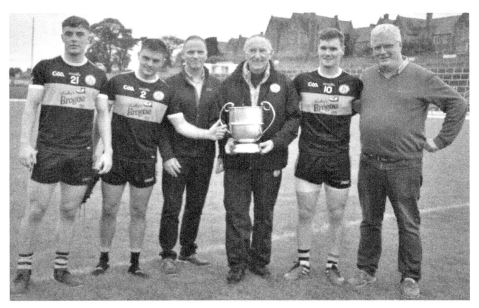

Armin Heinrich (21), Colin Griffin (2), Greg Horan (10), Eamon Whelan, Vice-Chairman Kerry GAA Board, third left, and former Austin Stacks Chairman Liam Lynch, right, join Billy Ryle, Austin Stacks Club Chairman, for a picture with the cup following the Senior Club Final victory in Killarney on 17th October 2021

CHAPTER THIRTY THREE

A DATE FOR CORNEAL TRANSPLANTATION

I travelled to Cork on the 12th October 2021 for my appointment with Mr Flynn. This was my first appointment since the 13th April 2021. During the six months between the visits, the sight in my right eye had deteriorated to such an extent that I felt sure that I needed surgery. Mr Flynn carefully examined both eyes and informed me that it was now reasonable to consider right corneal endothelial transplantation. In lay man's terms, the time was right to replace the inside layer of the cornea in my right eye with the inside layer from a donor cornea, whilst leaving the healthy parts of the cornea unaltered. This procedure would, hopefully, restore clarity in my right eye. We had discussed this procedure a number of times and I had carefully read Mr Flynn's printed information on the procedure. There was a very good chance that the procedure would improve the vision in my right eye. The risks involved were a dislocation of the graft which would require further surgery, glaucoma, graft failure and loss of vision from intraocular infection.

I was ready, willing and able for the corneal transplant to go ahead. More importantly, Mister Flynn was ready to do the operation. I was both excited by the prospect of improving my vision and apprehensive about having to go into Hospital to have the transplant done. But it was now or never and as I weighed up the positive outcomes against the negatives, the positive outcomes won hands down. Mr Flynn told me he would arrange a date for the corneal transplant and would let me know in due course. As I sat in the stand at the Fitzgerald Stadium on the following Sunday, 17th October, my resolve to go ahead with the procedure was redoubled. I struggled to follow the play and could only identify the players who came closest to me.

A few days later I received a letter from the Practice Co-ordinator with the admission details for my surgery with Mr Flynn. I would be admitted at 2.30pm on the 25th November 2021 at the Admissions Department, Bon Secours Hospital, College Road, Cork. I would be

required to stay one hight in Hospital. I was told that I would receive a
Local or General Anaesthetic. I was also reminded to ensure that I had
collected my post-operative medicines, which were eyedrops, as
prescribed by Mister Flynn and to bring them with me on the day of the
surgery.

I knew that the surgery would only proceed if I was fit and well. My
main concern was to avoid catching the Covid-19 Virus. I was also
determined to avoid flues, coughs, colds and any other infection which
might be in circulation at the time. I had diligently complied with the
HSE regulations since the first lockdown. I maintained my social
isolation and I avoided crowded situations in so far as I could. Éamonn
O Reilly, Austin Stacks Vice Chairman liaised with the senior football
mentors and players in his capacity as Coaching and Games
Development Officer. I avoided dressing rooms and team huddles and
all the other contacts that are fairly standard in football clubs. I observed
HSE protocols at our monthly meetings and at the other subcommittee
meetings which are part and parcel of the role of the Chairman of a big
football club.

 I also avoided the Club Bar, which meant that I missed a few
celebratory occasions throughout the season. I don't drink alcohol so I
was at no loss in that regard but I would like to have been in a position
to have shared in the post-match get-togethers with teams and club
members. I am a spiritual person who likes to attend Mass as regularly
as possible. No week passes when I don't manage to attend Mass on
three or four days. When the country was in lockdown, I took in Mass
on the RTE News channel and it was my intention to continue that
practice for the foreseeable future. My daily exercise was one of the
great pleasures in my daily routine. It served a dual purpose. It allowed
me to give my golden cocker spaniel dog, Jake, a decent walk and it
enabled me to enjoy my daily swim.

I prefer an early morning swim, so whenever there was sufficient tide at
Fenit bathing slip, Jake and I would drive back to the carpark in Fenit
around 8.45am. From there, we would walk along the path to the
swimming area where Jake would plonk down beside my clothes,

supposedly on guard duty but invariably asleep, while I enjoyed a refreshing dip in the salt water of the Atlantic Ocean. Then there was time for a chat and a cup of hot coffee with my swimming companions. I follow the tide all the time so I'd usually get about eight morning swims each fortnight while the other six were in the afternoon when the late tide had filled the bay.

As soon as I had received a definite date for my surgery, I had a chat with Éamonn O'Reilly, who was a great support to me not only as Club Chairman but also during the period when I was suffering with Fuchs Dystrophy. Éamonn and myself worked very well together and we became close friends during my term in office. I regularly approached him for advice and his informed views about issues that arose during our stewardship of Austin Stacks. He has an ideal temperament for leadership, a communication style that is respectful but decisive and a great capacity to get things done. In fact, he was an ideal wingman and I always knew Éamonn had my back when I needed a bit of rescuing, either from others or, indeed, from myself when I was planning to traverse some injudicious path. I often thought that he would have made a far better Chairman than myself and I sincerely hoped that when my three-year term as Chairman of Austin Stacks had expired, Éamonn would take over in the hotseat.

I informed Éamonn about the date of my surgery and that I would temporarily step aside as Austin Stacks Club Chairman if we were progressing in the Senior County Championship. If necessary, I would make the announcement at the November meeting of the Club Executive Meeting on Wednesday, 17th November 2021. I expected to be inactive for about four weeks and was hoping to have gotten the all-clear to resume normal service for the Club Executive meeting of Wednesday, 15th December 2021. I realised I would miss out on leading the club at County Senior Football Championship Semi-Final and Final stages if the team was fortunate enough to advance that far in the competition. I would of course attend the games in a more isolated part of the venues and I had full confidence in Éamonn's ability to represent the club with aplomb at the customary functions and events that are part and parcel of major football fixtures.

CHAPTER THIRTY FOUR

PROGRESS IN COUNTY SENIOR CHAMPIONSHIP

Sixteen teams went into the hat for the County Senior Football Championship draw. As luck would have it, Austin Stacks was paired with the holders East Kerry. Many Rock people were very disappointed with the draw, fearing that we would once again be eliminated in the first round of the County Championship. I felt from the start that any team with designs on winning the championship would have to beat East Kerry. While, on paper, the players available to the East Kerry manager were good enough to beat many county teams, Austin Stacks had two significant advantages at this early stage in the competition. Firstly, Austin Stacks was full of confidence after winning the Senior Club Championship a few weeks earlier. The team was battle hardened and playing great football. With so many club championship games at all levels taking place in the weeks before the senior county championship was due to commence, I was certain that the East Kerry squad would have done very little collective training. The time for East Kerry to prepare properly just wasn't there. The Divisional Board team hadn't played competitively together since the 2020 Kerry Senior Football Championship Final. The 2020 County Championship winners were at their most vulnerable against a team that had acquired the habit of winning games.

Our opening game in the County Senior Football Championship against East Kerry at Austin Stack Park at 7pm on Saturday, 30th October, 2021 was fixed as part of a double-header. The game was to be transmitted live on RTE 2. The opening game between St. Kierans and Kerins O'Rahillys would get underway at 5pm.

On a dreadful night in Austin Stacks Park, the champions looked lethargic from the get go. Our team hit the ground running and had fired over three points before East Kerry registered their only score, a point, before the first water break. We added two further points to a single point from East Kerry in the second quarter. At half time, The Rock led by five points to two and the team was playing out of its skin.

A similar pattern followed in the second half and with about ten minutes left in the game we led by 1-6 to 0-2. The champions were never going to relinquish the title without a fight and they threw everything at us in the concluding stages of the game. Seven additional minutes seemed like an eternity but our battle-hardened heroes held their ground and eliminated East Kerry from the 2021 County Senior Football Championship by 1-7 to 1-5. Austin Stacks progressed to the quarter-finals, which were pencilled in for the following weekend. We were now serious senior county championship contenders. No doubt, the other seven teams left in the competition felt the same way, now that the unbeatable East Kerry side had fallen by the way side. I knew that our squad of players would enjoy the victory over East Kerry but would keep their feet on the ground. They were experienced enough to know that the win in Round One would be quickly forgotten if we bit the dust in the next game.

The quarter finals quickly followed on the following weekend with a double header in Austin Stack Park on Saturday, 6th November featuring Dingle and Kerins O'Rahillys at 5pm and Legion and St. Brendans at 7pm. Then, on Sunday, 7th November in Fitzgerald Stadium, in a second double header, Templenoe would play Dr. Crokes at 12.45pm and Austin Stacks would take on South Kerry at 2.45pm. Once again, I was pleased to be facing a Divisional side that represented a huge geographical area. Now it was up to me to ensure that The Rockies, the famous club supporters, would travel in huge numbers to Killarney.

I made a direct and impassioned appeal directly to all Austin Stacks supporters to converge on Fitzgerald Stadium, Killarney and get behind our brilliant senior team in the quarter-final of the Garvey's Supervalu County Senior Football Championship against South Kerry. I continued – "The Stacks team is playing brilliant football and their spirited victory over East Kerry last Saturday night was a superb display of Rock football at its traditional best. Please travel to Killarney on Sunday to give your total backing to our team and mentors in their quest for victory in this vital game. Now is the time to show the rock-solid support for which Austin Stacks supporters are famous. Positive vocal encouragement from the 16th man on the terraces lets the players and mentors know that the Rockies are fully behind them. Your colourful and vocal presence in Tralee on Saturday night created the atmosphere that spurred-on our fearless warriors on the pitch. Austin Stacks is now one of the eight teams left in this prestigious competition. By 2.45pm on Sunday, The Rock will be one of the remaining five teams who can still win the Senior County Championship. Austin Stacks is determined to be in the semi-final draw on Sunday evening but we must defeat a very strong South Kerry team to achieve that aim. So, wear your black & amber colours with pride on Sunday and show your support for Manager Wayne Quillinan, his fellow mentors Mikey Collins, Jonathan Conway, Eoin Colgan, Tommy Naughton and John O Sullivan and our team squad, captained by the inspirational Dylan Casey, in their determination to progress to the semi-final of the Kerry Senior Football Championship. Your support on Sunday will be vital in continuing a wonderful journey for more senior silverware for Austin Stacks. C'mon the Rock! Na Stacaigh abú."

The Rock supporters took my call to arms to heart, as I expected them to do. The far terrace was a sea of black and amber just as it had been a few weeks before when we had won the Senior Club Championship. The Rockies had come to town and it wasn't to admire the natural landscape in 'Beauty's Home!'

By the time, South Kerry and Austin Stacks had taken the field on a pleasant dry day in Killarney, Kerins O'Rahillys, St. Brendans and Dr. Crokes had already qualified for the last four in the Kerry Senior Football Championship. Now, it was up to Austin Stacks to secure the fourth spot. From the throw-in, South Kerry looked a bit off of the pace and the score was 0-6 to 0-0 in our favour after the first fifteen minutes. The second quarter was more evenly balanced but we retained our six-point advantage to go in at half time leading by 0-9 to 0-3. With more of the same in the second half we would make it safely through to the semi-final.

That's exactly how it turned out except for a ten-minute period when South Kerry enjoyed a dominant spell during which they reduced the deficit to four points. But that was as good as it got for the Iveragh men as we added a further four points without reply to win by 0-14 to 0-6. Austin Stacks was through to the last four of the competition, which consisted of three club teams and a Divisional side.

For the third game in a row, it was our lot to draw the Divisional side, St Brendan's while the two other clubs, Kerins O'Rahillys and Dr. Crokes were destined to meet in the other semi-final. Our semi-final was fixed for 5.30pm on Saturday, 20th November at Austin Stack Park, Tralee and the second semi-final between Dr. Crokes and Kerins O'Rahillys would be played at 2.30pm on the following day at the same venue. RTE Television was showing our game live, but that didn't bother me unduly. There was no doubt in my mind that our supporters would flock to Austin Stack Park on the Saturday evening of the game.

About a week after the game with South Kerry, when I was preparing to temporarily step aside from my duties as Chairman and to pass the baton to my trusted Vice-Chairman, Éamonn O'Reilly, I received notification from The Elysian in Cork, that there wouldn't be a suitable donor organ available on the proposed date of my corneal transplant. It would be necessary to postpone my operation, which was scheduled to take place on Thursday, 25th November, 2021 at the Bon Secours Hospital, Cork to a date in the New Year. Initially I was shattered by this development as I had been building myself up psychologically for the procedure. Now I would have to stay in the zone until the transplant would be carried out in 2022.

On the other hand, perhaps the men of 1921, who brought the very first football title up Rock St., may have preordained that it was my destiny to lead Austin Stacks all the way to the Kerry Senior Football Championship title exactly one hundred years after that historic success in very troubled times. That thought gave me great consolation and peace of mind. My role now in the few weeks ahead would be to keep the momentum building for what lay ahead. I was confident that our team could win the on-field battles. I was also confident that I could win the psychological warfare that would surely take place off the field!

CHAPTER THIRTY FIVE

PENALTY SHOOT OUT IN SEMI-FINAL

As the build up to our semi-final with St Brendan's on Saturday, 20th November 2021 got underway, I found myself in an unusual situation. About thirty years earlier I had built a house in Spa village, which is about 5km from the town of Tralee. The location took me a few kilometres outside what would be considered natural Austin Stacks territory. As boundaries were no longer critical in deciding which club a player preferred to play with, I never thought too much about it. Austin Stacks had been in a number of county finals since I had settled in Spa village, but this semi-final was different as I was now Chairman of Austin Stacks and, because of the nature of the role, I had much more media profile. The ball hopping started earlier. Most of it was good natured banter where I gave as good as I got. The local Churchill GAA club would have players from Spa, Fenit and surrounding areas on the St Brendan's panel. My children would have attended Spa National school with some of them. I knew most of them personally and wished them well on the night, but, as a person who was born and reared in The Rock, Austin Stacks was always going to have my loyalty. All the more so on this occasion because as Club Chairman, I was the public face of the club and where ever I went in Tralee, Spa and Fenit the conversation was always dominated by the upcoming game.

The fact that Na Gaeil Club would be contributing a large contingent of players to the St Brendan's squad added another cutting edge to the semi-final. About forty years ago, Na Gael was founded in the Oakpark area of Tralee which was in the heartland of Austin Stacks territory. It left a lingering sting in the tale of Rock supporters. Tim Lynch Snr., who was Chairman of Na Gaeil Club for a number of years, is a personal friend of mine. We worked closely as Career Guidance Counsellors in neighbouring secondary schools in Tralee and you would travel a long way to find a more reasonable and considerate individual. Naturally, we often had a bit of banter before local derbies and the like. I always support a Tralee team when my own club is not involved so

Tim and I often exchanged good wishes before games. I fondly recall when I was on the road doing the Bracker 100km fundraising walk, Tim turned up to walk a stage of the journey with me. He even stood in for a photograph with me on the strict condition that it would never appear in public. I have respected his wish to-date but now that the book is hitting the shelves, who knows what might be included!

The semi-final game played under floodlights at Austin Stacks Park on Saturday evening, 20th November 2021 had everything you would expect from two superb teams and a lot more besides. It was tense from start to finish. After getting under way at 5.30pm the last kick was taken at 7.50pm, almost two and a half hours later. In all that time not one single spectator had left the Park. After a very even first half, the teams headed for the break having evenly shared six points. With about six minutes of normal time left to play the sides were still locked together at six points each. Then Michael O'Donnell finished the ball to the net for what looked like the decisive score for Austin Stacks. But this talented Divisional side was not giving up easily and, with nine minutes of agonising time added on, they managed to score the three points which resulted in a draw at the end of normal time on a score of Austin Stacks 1-6 to St. Brendan's 0-9. It was all to play for in extra time. Austin Stacks dominated the first period of extra time and seemed to have victory in sight when they led by 2-8 to 0-10 at the change-over. But this never-say-die St Brendan's side turned the tables around in that final period of extra-time by scoring 1-2 to our solitary point. The teams were still inseparable after extra -time. The final score was Austin Stacks 2-9 St Brendan's 1-12. This game was destined to be decided by a penalty shoot-out.

The penalty shoot-out was nerve racking but full of quality. All five Austin Stacks players scored and who else, but our star man Kieran Donaghy had the honour of dispatching the fifth and final penalty which sent our team into the County Senior Football Championship Final. This was the second penalty shoot-out success in a major senior competition during my stewardship. On my very first day as Chairman, Sunday, 15th December, 2019, Austin Stacks won the County Senior League, Division One title after a penalty shoot-out against Rathmore at the latter's venue. With Kerins O'Rahillys beating Dr Crokes in the second semi-final the scene was set for Tralee's El Clasico Kerry Senior Championship Final at Austin Stack Park on Sunday, 5th December. This would be the first meeting of the teams in the Kerry Senior Football Championship Final since 1936 and the town was a hub of excitement and anticipation.

On Monday night, 22nd November, 2021 just two nights after our semi-final victory, Éamonn O'Reilly and his Coaching Committee launched our new coaching manual. In his capacity as Coaching & Games Development Officer, Éamonn and his fellow members, Mike Casey, John O'Keeffe, Gene O'Donnell and Paudie McQuinn had taken on the task of producing a coaching manual that would incorporate the motto, mission, vision and values of Austin Stacks. It was a very enjoyable and informative night which was expertly facilitated by Éamonn and where well-prepared contributions were made by each of the authors of the document.

My role was primarily to provide the attendance with a short overview of the philosophy of Austin Stacks. I availed of the opportunity to welcome the coaching manual and to thank the Coaching Committee for providing the club with a document of pure quality. "The Coaching Committee," I added, "has devoted a considerable amount of time and effort in researching and writing a seminal reference manual while will enhance coaching standards throughout the club." I welcomed all of our team coaches and thanked them for their outstanding work with our playing members. "You are the lifeblood of Austin Stacks. Without our team coaches we wouldn't have teams. A special welcome to our female coaches tonight. This is a significant step towards the amalgamation of both our ladies and gents club," I said.

The launch of the Coaching Manual was a very special occasion for Éamonn O'Reilly and myself. All the heavy lifting had been done by Éamonn who brought coaching standards to a new level in the club. I was anxious for every coach to be up-to-speed on the style of play that should be developed up and down the club so that players could progress seamlessly up through the ranks to senior level. I was also anxious to have all coaching and management positions filled by our own members. That was the case at the time and I sincerely hoped that it would continue into the future.

In the weeks before a County Senior Football Final or a County Senior Hurling Final, its traditional that the clubs involved would host a media night at their club facilities. The players, in particularly, are in great demand for interviews and photographs. I saw the media night as an opportunity to showcase our club and the work that is ongoing throughout the club. Our media night took place on Tuesday, 23rd November 2021, the night after the very successful launch of our coaching manual. There was a fully representation of all the local press and media outlets. I saw my role as doing the formal introductions and words of welcome and then continuing in a more informal setting where our guests could speak individually with the players present. Later on, they could meet to speak with and or photograph our team mentors and playing squad who were training outside on our pitches. Along with myself at the top table were Wayne Quillinan, Dylan Casey and Kieran Donaghy. Éamonn O'Reilly, Club Vice-Chairman and Elma Nix, Club Secretary were all present as officers of the club and were available to interact with the press and media representatives.

I began by welcoming our guests in the build up to the County Senior Football Final. I continued by adding "The Rock Club is delighted to be in the final with Kerins O'Rahillys for the first time since 1936, now eighty-five years ago. Two of my maternal uncles Dan and Con Spring were members of the Kerins O'Rahillys team which lost out on that occasion to Austin Stacks by two points.

For the past few months our senior team has taken us on a magical journey by winning the Kerry Senior Club Championship for the third consecutive year and by defeating East Kerry, South Kerry and St Brendan's Divisional Boards on the way to the county final. In addition, our Senior B team went undefeated in the County Senior League, Division Five and went on win the final of that competition as well as gaining promotion to Division Four. That team also won their competition in the newly restructured Tralee & St Brendan's District Board.

Our total focus now is on bringing The Bishop Moynihan Cup back to Connolly Park on Sunday. We will succeed in doing that. Over the past few years. I have enjoyed watching the team go from strength to strength under the expert guidance of Wayne and his fellow mentors. I have never before met a team manager with the commitment and dedication of Wayne, who lets no stone unturned in his determination to win the Kerry Senior Football Championship. The Rock owes him a great deal of gratitude.

Our senior panel has had to put their lives, careers, studies and relationships on hold in order to reach the final. They are an exceptional group of young people who give their all for Austin Stacks. That will be good enough to make them county champions of Kerry on Sunday week.

Two great clubs, deep-rooted in GAA tradition will go head-to-head in this final. It's a mouth-watering prospect. Austin Stacks will be led out by our captain fantastic, the inspirational Dylan Casey, who has gone from being a good player to now being a great player.

If you are looking for the quintessential club player, look no further than Kieran Donaghy, who continues to give sterling service to his beloved Austin Stacks. His determination to win is infectious and will be a major factor in our success on Sunday week. What I admire most about Kieran is his unswerving loyalty to Austin Stacks. Despite his busy schedule Kieran is ever present on the team. He deserves another County Senior Football Championship winner's medal.

I'd like to mention especially my superb Vice-Chairman, Éamonn O'Reilly who doubles up as Coaching & Games Development Officer. While I have been concentrating on policy, administration, leadership and structures within the club, Éamonn closely liaises with Wayne and our three teams. We are very proud of our senior team and a totally united club is fully behind them.

The excitement, the anticipation, the craic is fever pitch around The Rock. Indeed, there is a festive atmosphere around the town. The game is bringing a welcome financial bonus to Tralee. Rock supporters are rushing out to purchase their black and amber colours. Let the entire town enjoy the pre-match razzamatazz. Let us celebrate this unique occasion of two Tralee town teams contesting the final. However, after the game on Sunday week, celebrations will be confined to Rocky territory as we welcome 'The Bishop' home."

The media night was very successful. Some of our players gave powerful interviews. My message to all members and supporters of the club was that while we greatly respected our opponents, we were quietly confident that this was our year to win the Kerry Senior Football Championship.

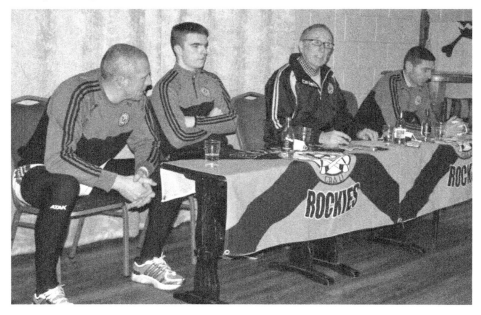

From left, Kieran Donaghy, Dylan Casey, Billy Ryle, Club Chairman and Wayne Quillinan, Team Manager were at the top table on the 23rd November 2021 for Austin Stacks Press Night prior to the Kerry Senior Football Championship Final

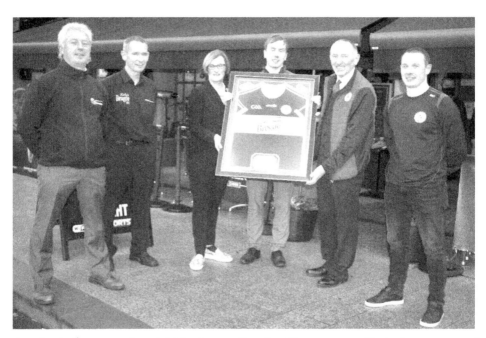

On the 25th November 2021, Austin Stacks Chairman Billy Ryle presented Fiona Cotter of Kirby's Brogue Inn, Club Sponsors, with a framed jersey prior to the Kerry Senior Football Championship Final. Pictured L/r: Éamonn O'Reilly, Vice- Chairman, Brian Morgan, Brogue Inn, Fiona Cotter, Shane O Callaghan, Senior Player, Billy Ryle and Mikey Collins, Senior Team Management

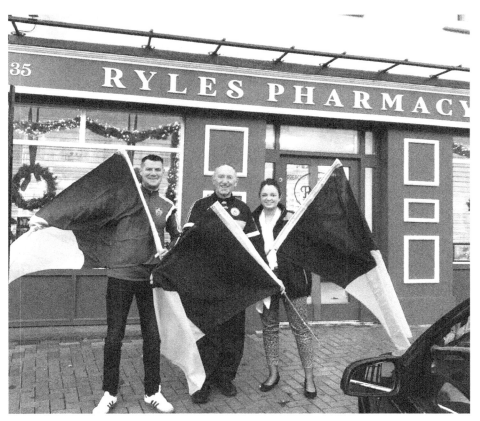

Billy Ryle pictured with his daughter Gráinne, supporting Austin Stacks and her business partner, Brian Daly, left, supporting Kerins O'Rahillys, on the build up to the 2021 Kerry Senior Football Championship Final at Austin Stack Park, Tralee.

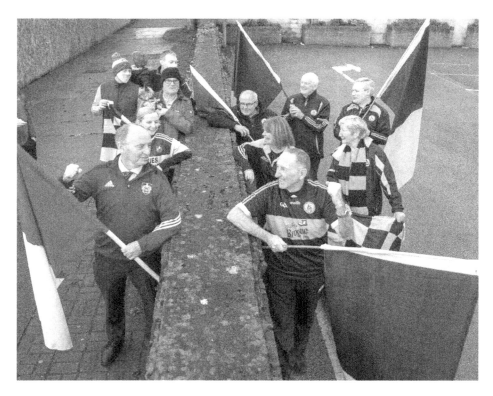

2021 Kerry Senior Football Final opponents meet at the dividing wall. On the Austin Stacks side are Billy Ryle, Mary Fitzmaurice, Mairéad Fernane, Paudie Commane, Jim Naughton and Shane Lynch. Kerins O'Rahillys Chairman, Haulie Kerins leads his troops on the other side.

CHAPTER THIRTY SIX

KERRY SENIOR FOOTBALL CHAMPIONS

In the two-week period, between the semi-final and the final, the members of the Club Executive Committee were very supportive and got fully behind the many preparations to be made and tasks to be done off the field. I delegated as much of the work as I could and my fellow members were very generous in their response. Each member had a particular skills-set and I saw the very best of them during the build-up to the final. I requested each member to be positive about our team but respectful of the opposition in conversation with media and with the public in general. The Executive Committee had been very progressive and diligent over the past few years. I was anxious for each one of them to share in a Kerry Senior Football Championship victory.

The local weekly papers were anxious to make the most of a local derby county final. On one occasion, I found myself in the town centre dressed in my club colours, holding a black & amber banner in one hand and waving the fist of my other hand at the Chairman of Kerins O'Rahilly's who was responding in kind. We had great craic and ball hopping as the public gathered around. The O'Rahilly's supporters who were present didn't believe me when I told them that everything was honkey-dory in our playing squad but rumour had it that a number of the O'Rahilly's players were carrying serious injuries. Similarly, for another photo shoot I was asked to have a few Rock supporters in the background. We turned up all decked out in black & amber and proudly waving our black and amber banners. A Strand Road man who was present felt a draw would be good for the town, which would have a second windfall on the day of a replay. "No chance of that happening," I quipped stoically, "Austin Stacks are going into the game to win it on the day," The psychological warfare was underway and it was a game I was very good at.

Similarly, when John O'Keeffe and myself did a pre-recorded interview for the TV company which was transmitting the game live, even the great Jonno smiled at the upbeat nature of my contribution. By the way, I never saw that interview as I had other things on my mind on the day! It was necessary to call a few extra meetings of the Club Executive Committee for review and updates. The feedback was very positive. All arrangements for the game had been finalised. Everything we could have done as an Executive Committee to smooth the path for our mentors and players had been done and done very well. It was time to play Kerins O'Rahilly in the 2021 Kerry Senior Football Championship Final.

The atmosphere around the town of Tralee in the days before the final on Sunday, 5th December was electric. The town centre was decorated with the colours of the competing teams. The Rock Street area of town was a sea of black and amber. It brought a tear to my eye. Final preparations were being put in place for the big parade from Connolly Park to the Austin Stack Park on Sunday. Thousands of Rock supporters marched down through the town in one of the most colourful parades witnessed before any county final. There was a taste of victory in the air. Now it was down to the players to perform on the day.

It was a cautious start by both sides. Nobody wanted to make a mistake or put in an ill-timed tackle that would result in a card being produced by the referee. After a quarter of an hour's play, the sides were level at three points each. We saw the best of our team in the second quarter as they slotted over five precious points to a single point in reply from Kerins O'Rahillys. We led by 0-8 to 0-4 at half time. Austin Stacks began the second half as they had finished the first half and we had a decent lead of 0-12 to 0-6 as we entered the final quarter of a game that was going according to plan. But O'Rahilly's threw caution to the wind and played their best football as the clock ticked down. The Blues slotted over four points against our solitary point. But our defence remained resolute and as we rapturously welcomed the sweet sound of the final whistle, Austin Stacks was ahead by 0-13 to 0-10. We were Senior Football Champions of Kerry for the first time since 2014. It was a fantastic feeling. My thoughts were drawn to the team which had won Austin Stacks first ever Kerry football title exactly one hundred years previously in 1921.

The pitch was invaded by elated Austin Stacks supporters. The exhausted but delighted players were surrounded by well-wishers issuing words of congratulations, back slapping and taking selfies with the players. It was a scene of joy unconfined. It was a proud moment for everybody associated with the Austin Stacks Club, for the playing squad and mentors and especially for Dylan Casey when he lifted the Bishop Moynihan Trophy. I stood on the pitch with Éamonn O'Reilly and said to him, "Well Éamonn, we have reached the Holy Grail after two years. We thought it might take three years but good leadership and the rub of the green has us here a year ahead of schedule."

I joined the Executive Committee, the winning team and mentors for a celebratory meal at the Brogue Inn Bar & Restaurant, our club sponsors. I was very pleased that we were able to deliver the Kerry Senior Football Championship title to Kevin and Fiona Cotter as repayment for the generous sponsorship that Éamonn O'Reilly and myself had negotiated with them two years earlier.

During the week, I extended my gratitude to all units of our great club for their generous contribution to our senior team's win in the Kerry Senior Football Championship Final. The huge level of support for the team, the indefatigable spirit, the unity of purpose, the all-time high morale in the club and the determination right across the club to pursue further success was heart-warming. I particularly acknowledged the 16th Man - the colourful, the noisy, the playful, the mischievous, the famous Rockie supporters.

"No other club is blessed with such loyal supporters. On Sunday, 19th December, 2021 we begin the next stage in the journey when we play Limerick champions, Newcastle West, in the Munster Senior Club Football Semi-final in Austin Stack Park at 1.30pm. This is a meeting of neighbouring County Champions so our gallant senior team will need the same level of support that spurred our team on to victory in the county final. So, Austin Stack supporters, once again on Sunday, 19th December convert the far terrace into a sea of black and amber. Let the drums roll out and let the flags fly proudly in the wind. Let the Rockie anthems rent the seasonal air. The stakes are very high with a place in the Munster Senior Club Football Final in the New Year up for grabs. As a united and focussed Club, Austin Stacks can achieve that place in the final," I added.

As expected, Austin Stacks had a reasonably comfortable victory over Newcastle West, Limerick in the semi-final of the Munster Senior Club Football Championship which was played at Austin Stack Park, Tralee on Sunday, 19th December 2021. After a very accomplished performance we led by 0-9 to 0-1 at half time. As the gap increased to 1-13 to 0-5 in the second half, the Manager was able to run his bench. Final score was 1-15 to 0-8 in favour of Austin Stacks. We were in the Munster Senior Club Football Final which would be played early in 2022.

At the final meeting of the Executive Committee the following Tuesday night, 21st December 2021, a Steering Group was set up to direct the off-the-field support activities for our senior team in the build up to the Munster Final which we now knew would be played on Sunday, 16th January, 2022. The Steering Group would be informal and activity based. All Executive members were invited onto the group which would concentrate on logistics and planning events up to and including match day. Fundraising would be outside the brief of the Steering Group as our Treasurers were working with an experienced team of fundraisers and they would update us, as appropriate.

I, as Club Chairman, would coordinate the activities of the Steering Group and provide regular updates for all members of the Executive Committee, whether or not they joined the Steering Group. So, I requested my colleagues to run any information and ideas they may have by me - approaches about one off sponsorships, requests to guest on a podcast, events happening, etc, - and I would circulate the collective information every few days. I stated that it was my hope that all of us would be prepared to share in the various functions, duties and tasks that would promote and maintain the momentum behind our team. Our Steering Group, I added, could go a long way to fostering the feel-good factor, the positivity, the unity, the spirit and the sense of purpose that was very evident in Austin Stacks and Tralee at present. I stated that it would be necessary to call a few meetings at short notice – relaxed, informal, action based, updating, planning ahead and task allocation.

The response from my colleagues was very positive. I was very pleased that we now had a Steering Group and a Fundraising Team in place before Christmas to assist our senior team in winning the Munster Senior Club Football Championship.

As we approached the end of a very successful year both on and off the field, my final duty of 2021 was to extended season greetings to Austin Stacks members and supporters and to request their continuing support in 2022.

As Club Chairman, I extended warm season's greetings to Rock people at home and abroad. I wished club members and supporters everywhere a very happy Christmas and good health in the New Year. I extended sincere thanks to everybody, who served Austin Stacks in any capacity during the year as administrators, team officials, volunteers and players.

"We all rejoiced in the wonderful successes which Austin Stacks achieved during the past twelve months. Pride of place goes to our senior team which won the Kerry Senior Football Championship exactly 100yrs after The Rock Street Club won it's very first county football title, the Kerry Junior Football Championship, in 1921. The Club won the first of its thirteen Kerry Senior Football Championships in 1928, captained by the great Joe Barrett.

Our resolute senior team has now qualified for the Munster Senior Club Football Championship Final against St. Finbarr's, Cork in mid-January 2022. Let's begin the New Year by winning that prestigious title. Our great club will be relying on the famous Rockie supporters to rally behind the team in the final. I am appealing to Austin Stacks supporters everywhere to attend the final and convert the venue into a sea of black and amber. As a united, determined and focussed club, Austin Stacks will win this final.

Club members can play an important part in the ongoing development and successes of the club at all levels by taking on an active role in administration and team mentoring at whatever level they feel comfortable. Supporters can best serve the club by becoming paid-up members in 2022. Membership fees are an important source of club income.

I am encouraging all members to actively participate in the Austin Stack Club Annual General Meeting on the 23rd January 2022. Nominations for all positions on the Club Executive Committee will be accepted from this week. Please make yourself available to serve on the Club Executive Committee or on any of the subcommittees which ensure that Austin Stacks is run efficiently and to the highest standards.

Please stay safe and well during the holiday period and continue to comply fully with Government and GAA health guidelines to ensure that our members and their families are protected from the deadly omicron virus. Beannachtaí na Nollag oraibh go léir," I said.

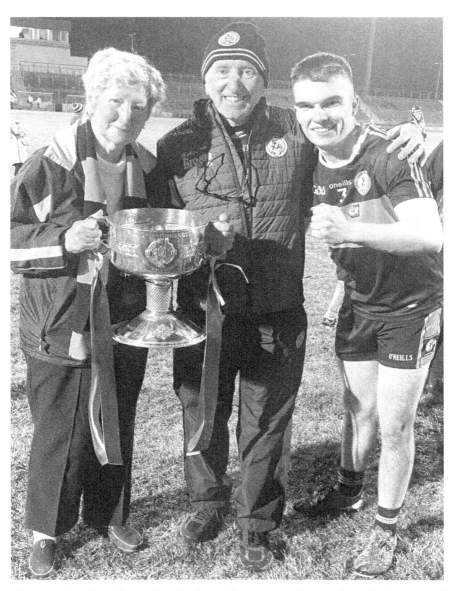

Austin Stacks Captain, Dylan Casey is pictured with Mairéad Fernane and Billy Ryle and, of course, The Bishop Moynihan Cup after the Kerry Senior Football Championship Final on Sunday, 5th December 2021.

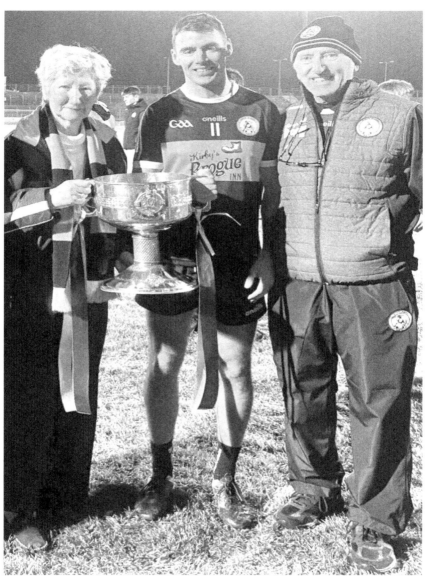

Austin Stacks player Fiachna Mangan poses for a picture with Mairéad Fernane and Billy Ryle after the victory over Kerins O'Rahillys in the 2021 Kerry Senior Football Championship final on the 5th December 2021.

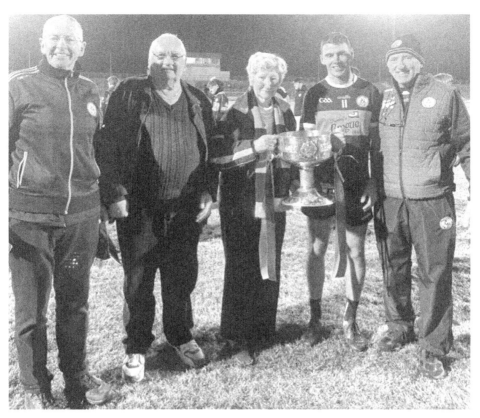

Fiachna Mangan lines up for a photo with, from left, his proud father, Colm, Tim Guiheen, Mairéad Fernane and Billy Ryle after the victory over Kerins O'Rahillys in the 2021 Kerry Senior Football Championship Final on the 5th December 2021.

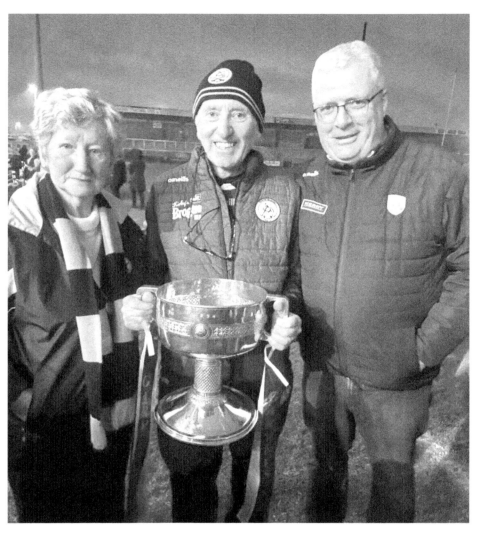

Three proud Chairpersons of Austin Stacks, Mairéad Fernane, Billy Ryle and Liam Lynch are pictured with The Bishop Moynihan Cup after the Kerry Senior Football Championship Final on Sunday, 5th December 2021.

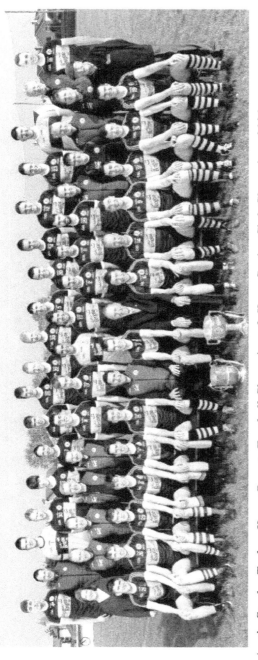

Austin Stacks, Tralee: Kerry County Football Champions & Kerry Senior Club Champions 2021

Front Row L/r - Luke Chester, Donagh McMahon, Jordan Kissane, Michael O'Gara, Ronan Shanahan, Darragh O'Brien, Wayne Quillinan (Team Manager), Dylan Casey (Team Captain), Billy Ryle (Club Chairman), Conor Jordan, Kieran Donaghy, Greg Horan, Dara Barry Walsh, Ciarán O'Connell, Seán Quilter.

Middle Row L/r – Elma Nix (Club Secretary), Kieran Shannon, Eoin Colgan, Jonathan Conway, Damien Ryall, Joseph O'Connor, Shane O'Callaghan, Wayne Guthrie, Barry Shanahan, Colin Griffin, Fiachna Mangan, Gearóid Fitzgerald, Fionnan Hallinan, Matthew Browne, Tommy Naughton, John O'Sullivan, Martin Collins (Club PRO).

Back Row – Jack O'Shea, Mikey Collins, Ben Quilter, Gearóid Sheehan, Cian Purcell, Andrew Morrissey, Armin Heinrich, David Fitzmaurice, Barry Walsh, Joey Nagle, Paul O'Sullivan, Adam Curran, Niall Fitzmaurice, Brendan O'Sullivan, Jack Morgan, Robbie Murphy, Éamonn O'Reilly (Club Vice-Chairman), Michael O'Donnell

Photo courtesy of Martin Cleary

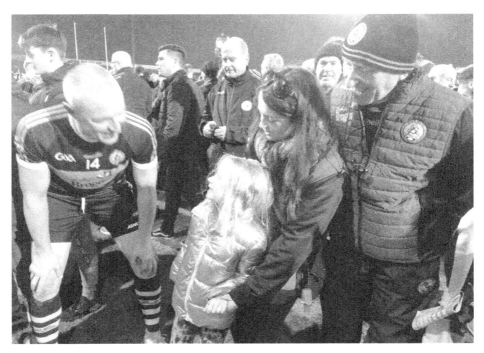

Kate Ryle congratulates her star man, Kieran Donaghy, after the 2021 Kerry Senior Football Championship win at Austin Stack Park on 5th December 2021 as Gráinne and Billy Ryle, Club Chairman, enjoy the moment

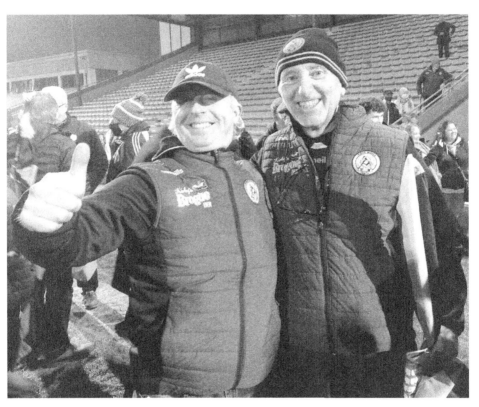

We've done it! Éamonn O Reilly and Billy Ryle in great form after the Kerry Senior Football Championship win at Austin Stack Park on 5th December 2021

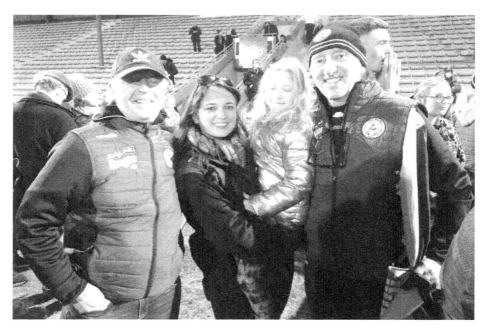

Éamonn O Reilly, left, celebrates with Gráinne, Kate and Billy Ryle after Austin Stacks win in the 2021 Kerry Senior Football Championship on the 5th December 2021.

CHAPTER THIRTY SEVEN

PSYCHOLOGICAL WARFARE

During the three weeks between Christmas Day 2021 and Sunday, 16th January 2022, which was the day fixed for the Munster final, Austin Stacks was a hive of activity. Both our Steering Group and our Fundraising Team, respectively, were meeting regularly and making great progress. I was anxious to have a venue for the game pinned down before Christmas so that our Steering Group could press ahead with travel arrangements for our team and supporters. According to the regulations this game had to be played at a neutral venue unless the teams agree to toss a coin for home venue. I firmly expected that the game would be played at the Gaelic Grounds, Limerick. The trip to Limerick would be very convenient for both teams and the facilities in Limerick were first rate.

On Monday, 20th December 2021, I was contacted by an official of Munster GAA, who informed me that Limerick GAA Board and Tipperary GAA Board were not keen to make Limerick Gaelic Grounds and Semple Stadium, Thurles, respectively, available for the game. I was taken aback by this information as this game, along with the equivalent hurling final, is the most prestigious fixture in the Munster club competitions calendar. The official asked me if Austin Stacks would agree to toss a coin for a home fixture in Austin Stack Park, Tralee or Páirc Uí Rinn, Cork. I requested some time to consult with fellow club officials and was asked by the Munster GAA official to submit Austin Stacks decision by 6pm that afternoon.

I replied before 6pm stating that Austin Stacks would be very happy to toss a coin for home venue in order to assist the Munster GAA in its difficulty in acquiring a venue and because Austin Stacks would have a 50/50 chance of bringing this attractive fixture to Tralee. It would also mean that, in the precarious times of virulent delta and omicron pandemic variants, the supporters of only one of the two clubs involved would have to travel.

The prospect of playing the game in Tralee on the 16th January 2022 was very attractive to Austin Stacks. The famous Rockie supporters would bring their customary carnival razzamatazz and good humour to the occasion. The atmosphere in Austin Stack Park would be electric with the black and amber colours blowing proudly in the wind, with the drums beating loudly and the Stack's supporters in full voice. The home fixture would also give Tralee a huge financial boost and a feel-good factor in the build-up to the game. The whole town was backing The Rock in this fixture. Playing the game in Austin Stack Park would be our way of giving something back to our beloved town in terms of a welcome spending spree and a great buzz of anticipation about the place.

If the toss went against us, Austin Stacks would look forward to a great spectacle in Páirc Uí Rinn, which would be invaded by our loyal supporters. I was sure our supporters would outnumber the home support and I was confident that our gallant team would beat St. Finbarr's in their own backyard. Alas! The Munster GAA official informed me early on Tuesday morning, 21st December, 2021 that St. Finbarr's were not prepared to toss for home venue and were insisting on a neutral venue. I was taken aback by their rejection of an opportunity to have the game played in Cork. Or perhaps, they were running scared of The Rock and not prepared to risk the game being played in Tralee!

I informed the Munster GAA official that, in that event, Austin Stacks would prefer to play the final at the Gaelic Grounds, Limerick but that we would have no problem in going to Thurles if Munster GAA so decreed. Since Tuesday, 21st December, I was to-and-fro with Munster GAA. In my final communication with Munster GAA about 5pm on Thursday, 23rd December, I was informed – and I quote – "we don't have anything confirmed yet. The Gaelic Grounds and Semple Stadium won't commit at the moment. The management committee will meet on the 4th January 2022 to try and tie the details down." I was concerned by the lack of urgency in that statement which confirmed that no decision would be taken about the venue before the 4th January 2022, at the earliest, nine working days before the game was due to be played. Austin Stacks needed adequate time to put the normal logistical arrangements in place. We needed to know where the game was going to be played. This was a very big game for The Rock, Tralee and Kerry, so I wanted to avoid any procrastination and indecision during the week beginning 4th January which could have resulted in a venue for the game not been decided until the eleventh hour.

I left Austin Stacks' offer to toss a coin for home venue on the table and in the spirit of the Christmas season, I requested St. Finbarr's to reconsider their refusal to help out Munster GAA in its present difficulty. It's was a great opportunity to keep the game local for one of the teams. Tralee or Cork would get a much-needed financial fillip. If St. Finbarr's won the toss, Austin Stacks would look forward to playing them and beating them in Páirc Uí Rinn on the 16th January. Alternatively, if Austin Stacks won the toss, we would look forward to playing The Barrs in Tralee where they would be guaranteed the best of hospitality in the friendliest town in Ireland.

St. Finbarr's were resolute in their refusal to toss for home venue and the game was fixed for 1.45pm in Semple Stadium, Thurles on Sunday, 16th January 2022. When asked for a reaction to the choice of venue, I stated that "Austin Stacks Club is delighted that the AIB Munster Senior Club Football Championship Final has been fixed for 1.45pm on Sunday, 16th January 2022 at Semple Stadium, Thurles, which is the second largest GAA Stadium in Ireland. The spectacular Semple Stadium in Thurles is an ideal choice to host a game of this significance and Austin Stacks is looking forward to meeting St Finbarr's at a venue with a superb atmosphere, top class facilities and a wonderful pitch, which will facilitate a game of top-class football.

Our resolute senior team, which has taken us on a wonderful journey this season – Kerry Senior Club Championship and Kerry Senior

Football Championship successes - is thrilled to have qualified for the Munster Senior Club Football Championship Final against St. Finbarr's. The Rock, Tralee and Kerry is backing Austin Stacks to win this prestigious title on Sunday week. It might be a long way to Tipperary, but our famous Rockie Army – the 16th Man – will rally behind the team in the final. I am confident that Austin Stacks supporters everywhere will arrive in huge numbers into Thurles by train, bus and car to attend the final and to convert the venue into a colourful display of black and amber. As a united, determined and focussed club, Austin Stacks are coming to town to win this coveted title."

The first phase in the customary pre-match psychological warfare was now over. I was pleased to have won that skirmish. St Finbarr's had been put on the defensive. They were the team unprepared to toss for venue. In response, I knew in my heart and soul that every Rock supporter would make an extra special effort to be in Thurles on the 16th January. We had less than two weeks to get them there.

I convened a meeting of our Steering Group on Wednesday, 5th January 2022 to share our feed-back and to firm up our arrangements. Semple Stadium, Thurles was confirmed as venue for the game. The most feasible transport would be checked out immediately – an excursion trained was preferred but coaches were also an option. Supporters' leaders would be kept in the loop about transport plans in order to aid coordination. Suitable venues in Thurles would be checked out as the supporters' base – refreshments and lunch, etc. - and the gathering point for the parade to the stadium. Éamonn O'Reilly would touch base with the team management to exchange information in order to aid the coordination of preparation. There was good news about sponsorship of a new set jerseys for the senior panel. There was excellent news from The Brogue Inn Bar & Restaurant that our agreed sponsorship would be extended for an extra year and that bonus payments would be provided to defray some of the cost of the current senior campaign. I agreed to meet with Stephen Stack, Manager AIB, Tralee to check if complimentary tickets would be available to Austin Stacks for the Munster final and to discuss a possible financial contribution for

Munster final expenses. I also agreed to contact Munster GAA regarding ticket sales and club ticket allocation, etc.

It was a vibrant meeting and I was delight by the enthusiasm and the good will on show from those in attendance. I felt that no stone would be left unturned by these fine people in their efforts to help our team win the Munster title. The feed-back was so prominent during the days that followed that I was able to issue an update to the Steering Group on Saturday, 8th January, 2022.

Stephen Stack would very kindly provide complimentary match tickets on behalf of the competition sponsors, but as AIB was the national sponsor of the Club Championship, a local financial contribution would not be possible. Great progress had been made in arranging coach transport to Thurles as Irish Rail was not in a position to provide a special train due to the Covid-19 pandemic. Representatives of the supporters were briefed about possible travel arrangements and were pleased to liaise with us in finalising arrangements. Éamonn has spoken with Wayne Quillinan and both have exchanged up-to-date information. Éamonn would update the Steering Group at our next meeting. Éamonn had provisionally arranged for Hayes' Hotel in Thurles to be our base for refreshments and food, etc., and gathering point for the parade. I had spoken to Munster GAA. Austin Stacks would receive a ticket allocation which, when added to the AIB allocation, would be sufficient to cover our ticket requirements for our team, support team and sponsors.

Online tickets for the match could be purchased from the following week. The Club would also assist supporters who were unable to purchase online tickets, with ticket purchase, as tickets would not be available for purchase at the venue. I stated that I would convene a meeting of the Steering Group as soon as the transport arrangements were firmed up.

Logistics were falling nicely into place. Our Steering Group met for the final time before the final on Wednesday, 12th January. We were happy that all the logistics were in place for Sunday. All the complimentary tickets were prepared for distribution. We were informed that the Fundraising Team had been very successful in raising money. A 'Go fund me' page had been set up and donations were being made. The supporters' buses were organised and the supporters' leaders had all the arrangements made for the big parade from our base at Hayes' Hotel to Semple Stadium. The players and mentors were travelling up on Saturday to a hotel outside of Thurles.

I must admit that I had some misgivings about the overnight stay in Tipperary. I would have preferred the players to have slept in their own beds the night before the game. Many of our players were young and might have been more relaxed in the bosom of their families. The journey to Thurles from Tralee is relatively short and I expected that we would arrange for the players to travel up in cars with family or club officials or else in a team bus. The psychological implications of the players trying to pass the time in unfamiliar surroundings on Saturday evening and Sunday morning caused me some unease. However, as the arrangements had been finalised and everybody seemed to be happy with them, I didn't verbalise my misgivings. The unity and sense of purpose throughout all sections of the club was very strong and I was determined to maintain the momentum for the game. I, myself, would be unable to travel on the Saturday before the final for an overnight stay in a hotel due to my Fuchs Dystrophy. With surgery scheduled for early in the New Year it was necessary for me to social distance and avoid infection or illness that would cause the postponement of my operation.

CHAPTER THIRTY EIGHT

NEW DATE FOR SURGERY

While the preparations for the Munster Final were in full swing, I received notification from Cork that my right eye corneal transplant operation, which had been postponed on Thursday, 25th November 2021 had been rescheduled for Thursday, 10th February 2022. I was expecting a date for my procedure and I suppose I was relieved when it came. The quality of the vision in my right had deteriorated considerably and I had a slight haze in the vision in my left eye. If I could get the corneal transplant in my right eye, I would, hopefully, have improved vision in that eye. All going well, I was sure that, later in the year, Mr Flynn would perform cataract surgery and, subsequently, a corneal transplant operation in my left eye. It looked like I would be heading to the Bon Secours Hospital, Cork for at least three surgical procedures during the coming year. I would also have to travel to Cork for regular appointments with Mr Flynn. I thought about the implications of my Fuchs Dystrophy and made the tough decision that my sight would have to be my primary concern for the coming year.

It had been my intention to serve for three years as Chairman of Austin Stacks. I have a great affection for the club and I was very pleased with the leadership I had brought to the club during the previous two years. Of course, I had some unfinished business. The Munster and All-Ireland Senior Club Football Championship titles were still to be won. There was no doubt in my mind that Austin Stacks had the strongest team left in these competitions. I had been lucky that Austin Stacks had won so much silverware during my term of office. I wanted that karma to continue all the way to Croke Park. As our Annual General Meeting wasn't due until Sunday, 23rd January 2022, I would still be Chairman for the Munster final on Sunday, 16th January, but with profound regret and after much soul searching, I made the decision not to seek re-election at the AGM.

At the time, I was the only nominee for the position of Chairman, but I was confident that Éamonn O'Reilly would be prepared to succeed me in the position. As I mention, Éamonn and I had a very warm and productive working relationship as the two most senior officers in the Club. Most of the three-year development plan that we used to talk about had been implemented in two years and Austin Stacks was now the super club that we wanted it to be. The Munster final trophy would be my last hurrah and Éamonn would lead the club to All-Ireland glory. No man was more deserving of that honour.

With a heavy heart, I emailed to the Club Secretary that I had been called for a corneal transplant operation in my right eye in early February. Consequently, I regretted that I would not be a candidate for the position of Club Chairman at the AGM on Sunday, 23rd January, 2022. I also, as a matter of courtesy, followed up with an email to each member of the Club's Executive Committee informing them that I had been called for a corneal transplant operation in my right eye in early February and that I would have to isolate before the surgery and avoid post-operative infection, which could cause rejection of the organ, for a few months.

"I have informed the Club Secretary that I will not be a candidate for the position of Club Chairman at the AGM on Sunday, 23rd January, 2022. It was a great privilege to serve as Club Chairman for the past two years but it's now necessary for me to step aside and make way for the appointment of a new Chairman at the AGM.

I will continue to fulfil the duties of Chairman to the best of my ability until the incoming Chairman takes office on 23rd January. My main focus will be on facilitating our senior team's victory in the Munster Senior Football Championship Final on the 16th January and, in my final week as Chairman, preparing for the AGM. I'm confident that my successor can lead the team to All-Ireland success.

The club has enjoyed considerable achievements on the field of play during the past two years. Each of you will have your own cherished memories. For me, it was that very special day in Castleisland when our

Senior B team won Division Five of the Kerry Senior League. I felt very proud of the team and mentors on that particular day but especially of Paddy Barry whose dignity and resilience in the face of an incalculable personal loss during the year made a lasting impression on me.

I will play no part in the appointment of the next Chairman. However, I feel that it would be in the best interests of Austin Stacks if a member of the outgoing Executive Committee was to take on the chairmanship in order to provide continuity in the great work we shared together.

Finally, when Austin Stacks came calling two years ago, I am glad that I answered the call. I always felt that I owed a debt of service to a Club which gave me a value system that sustained me through a very fulfilling life. That debt has now been paid. As a loyal and proud Rockie, I look forward to supporting our teams from the anonymity of the terraces and in helping out on one or two subcommittees, if required. With warmest regards and God's Blessing on each of you in 2022," I added.

I was surprised and disappointed when Éamonn O'Reilly decided not to become my successor as Chairman. I respected his decision as I know that he carries a great deal of responsibility in his day job. However, I was delighted that he was remaining on as Vice-Chairman. When Shane Lynch was nominated for the position, I was certain that the club would be in safe hands going forward. Shane had been very helpful to Éamonn and myself when we went in search of sponsorship early in 2020. It was Shane who prepared the package which we presented to potential sponsors as we tried to put the Club on a sound financial footing. It was a very attractive package which impressed those with whom we discussed it. Shane has such a forensic understanding of the world of finance that it makes him invaluable to Austin Stacks. I was very pleased that he accepted my invitation to join the Executive Committee in January 2021. He was a breath of fresh air and brought a great deal of energy, ability and creativity to the Executive. He had the skills-set and the work ethic to become a very successful Chairman of Austin Stacks where he has deep roots.

On Tuesday, 11th January, 2022, the night before the final meeting of the Steering Group, the Annual General Meeting of our Juvenile Club took place. I have always been convinced that our Juvenile Club is the jewel in the crown of Austin Stacks. Not only is it a conveyer belt for our minor and senior teams, but the calibre of the mentors guarantees that our young players require a skills-set and value system that serves them well on the journey through life. As Club Chairman, I felt it was important during my term of office that I should regularly pay tribute to the those who were doing such outstanding work in the under-age section of our great Club. 2021, just like the previous year, had been a very difficult year because of the playing restrictions imposed by the coronavirus. Nevertheless, a great deal had been achieved both on and off the field.

Year after year, our Juvenile officers and team mentors do outstanding work with our young members. They give our youngsters a great start in life through imparting a value system, which includes ambition, loyalty, self-discipline, team work, a sense of community, a work ethic and, of course, a lifelong affection for Austin Stacks. They expose the youngsters to the skills of the game, the joy of training and playing the game and whatever competitive success it brings as they progress through the various age ranks. They provide a conveyor belt of footballers right up to senior level, many of whom go on to achieve great things with Austin Stacks and Kerry.

Our club mentors at all levels deserve great credit for the success which the club attains in all its competitions. Our Juvenile Club is accustomed to regular success through all its age groups and that will continue in the years ahead. But those involved in our Juvenile Club, like myself as Club Chairman, know that building a successful senior team is a long-term project which begins on the very first day the youngsters arrive at the Academy. Our juvenile mentors nurture these young people through the years and every so often a dream team emerges to win a Senior County Championship and, on occasion, a Munster and All-Ireland title. Our entire cohort of under-age mentors deservedly share in and can be very proud of the successes of our senior teams.

As mentioned earlier, in 2021 Austin Stacks launched a three-year sponsorship with Ned O'Shea Construction Ltd and John Lane & Sons Ltd, Food Service Distribution, who were jointly sponsoring Austin Stacks U-17, U-15 and U-13 teams – six teams in total – from 2021 to 2023, inclusive. On behalf of our Juvenile Club, as we began a new year, it was appropriate that I should extend sincere thanks to Benny Murphy and Pat Lane who structured a three-year financial plan for the under-age teams involved.

Through the O'Shea/Lane sponsorship we established a formal working relationship with Jigsaw Kerry, which is a free mental health support service for young people. The jerseys of the six sponsored teams are displaying the logo, Jigsaw Kerry Youth Mental Health and Austin Stacks is availing of the expertise of Jigsaw Kerry to provide mental health information, support and counselling for our young players. This great service, which is a new departure in a GAA Club, was structured by Mike Casey on behalf of Austin Stacks and Frank O'Rahilly of Jigsaw Kerry, who deserve great credit for a unique accomplishment.

One of the highlights for me during 2021 was the production of the excellent coaching manual by our Coaching Committee. This is a very valuable document which not only includes a detailed coaching manifesto but also the mission, vision and values of our club. The chosen motto – TEAM – Together Everybody Achieves More – couldn't be more appropriate. Austin Stacks is a Club where the TEAM ethic is very strong and that is why the Club achieves so much at all levels. The coaching manual has been a huge addition to the quality of information available to our coaching, mentoring and administrative staff and will be very beneficial to the general membership as the Club continues to build for the future.

As the new year began, I wished the Juvenile Club a successful and, hopefully, an uninterrupted 2022. I expressed my gratitude to all of our members who were taking on duties as administrators and team officials during 2022. As well as the great work our mentors do with the young players, I know that they enjoy the training and the games, the friendships they make and the on-field successes their young teams achieve during the year.

Following a very industrious meeting of the Munster Final Steering Group on the following evening, the final few days were spent in crossing the t's and dotting the i's of our detailed preparation for our trip to Tipp! All roads now let to Semple Stadium for the showdown with St. Finbarr's.

CHAPTER THIRTY NINE

THE DREAM DIES IN THURLES

On a fine sunny morning on Sunday 16th January 2022, my wife and I set out for Thurles. It was a very pleasant trip with a steady flow of cars flying black and amber flags heading in the same direction as ourselves. The buses carrying supporters had set out directly from our club premises in Connolly Park, Tralee. Thurles was a hive of excitement as we drove past Semple Stadium, which was beginning to show signs of activity. It had been some since we had last attended a game in Thurles and the sight of the magnificent grounds increased our anticipation. This pitch always evoked happy memories of the wonderful point that Maurice Fitzgerald slotted over the crossbar from an impossible angle for Kerry again the Dubs while Tommy Carr was doing his best to distract Maurice. They were great memories and we were confident that more good memories would be made on that special Sunday.

We were early so we drove past the venue and continued into the town centre to soak up the atmosphere and link up with our friends. There was a very convenient carpark close to Hayes Hotel so we availed of it along with other Rock supporters who were arriving around the same time. We decided to have a meal immediately and headed for Hayes Hotel. There was a queue out the door and it was moving very slowly. The wait for seating would take far too long so we drifted down the street and found a nice Restaurant. There were some vacant tables and most of the diners were either Austin Stacks or St. Finbarr's supporters. The banter was warm and friendly. We chatted with some Cork people, who were confident that St. Finbarrs would win. They were a family of two parents and three young children who were very excited about being in Thurles to support their team. I hadn't the heart to spoil their day at this early stage so I replied, "We'll do our best to give ye a good game, but it's not easy beat the Rebels." "Up the Barrs, boy, up the Barrs like," the children replied in unison. We wished them well and made a timely exit. I was hoping that we would not bump into them after the game when the disappointment of defeat would be etched on their little faces!

We made our way back to the square where the Rockie supporters were congregating in large numbers. All the loyal regulars were present. There were also unfamiliar faces, some of whom were attending their first game of the season. I was glad to welcome them all. There is an old saying that success has many parents but that failure is an orphan. That may be true but, from my perspective, every supporter counted. The more supporters Austin Stacks would have during this final the merrier as far as I was concerned. Our 16th Man had often got us over the line in tight situations. Each and every one of them had a role to play in achieving victory. The parade was wonderful to behold. The main street of Thurles was converted into a sea of black and amber. The mighty drums rolled out and the Rock banners flew majestically in the early spring sunshine. Our battle anthems rent the air. We had fire in our bellies. The Rockies were on the march to Semple Stadium with a definite mission to cheer their heroes to victory. The supporters were worth their weight in gold.

My wife, Sheila and I made our way to the seats that would afford me the best possible vantage point. We found excellent seats towards the front of the stand, midway between the goal posts. The section of the stand directly behind us was packed with Austin Stacks supporters. Immediately, I realised I had a problem. The strong low-lying sun was shining directly in my face. The sun was setting in the west while we were looking straight at it from the east. I would have to make the best of it and rely on my wife and those around me for information. By putting my hand over my eyes, I was able to follow the play on the near side of the pitch but saw very little on the far side.

The tenson was palpable as the teams warmed up and went through the pre-match formalities. This would be my last game as Chairman of Austin Stacks. The year 2021 had been an "Annus Mirabilis" for me in terms of winning silverware. I was very anxious to bow out with the Munster Senior Club Football Championship trophy. Shane could then lead The Rock through two more games to the All-Ireland Senior Club Football Championship title.

St Finbarrs shook us with a goal directly from the throw-in. Austin Stacks was rattled. The team was flatfooted and lethargic. What was wrong. We urged them to settle down. We knew they were a good team but had the occasion gotten to them? It was early in the game. They had plenty of time to get to grips with the speed of the action. It didn't happen in the first half which belonged to the Cork team. They were fast and aggressive. They constantly attacked when possession came their way. They were by far the better team in the first half and went in at the break leading by 1-7 to our 0-4.

I'd like to have been a fly on the wall in the Austin Stacks dressing room during the interval. Whatever was said certainly worked the oracle. We saw the real Austin Stacks in the first quarter of the second half. This was the form that we had so admired during the county championship campaign. This was more like the fighting spirit that had turned games in our favour. The Cork team was now on the backfoot. They failed to score in the third quarter while The Rock added on five precious points. It was 1-7 to 0-9 at the second water break. We were back in the game and getting stronger as the game progressed.

The Barrs extended their lead to two points on the resumption. In the last minute of normal-time they got through for a second goal to stretch their lead to five points. Leading by 2-8 to 0-9 they looked home and hosed. But our gallant players didn't throw in the towel. Throwing caution to the wind, they attacked with purpose to score a pointed free followed by a magnificent goal. A single point separated the teams. On this occasion lady luck deserted us and the Cork team scored the final point of the game to take the title by two points. Final score was St. Finbarr's 2-9 Austin Stacks 1-10.

Our dream of a Munster Senior Club Football Championship title died on the green sod of Semple Stadium. Our season had ended and so would my term as Club Chairman on the following Sunday. Our team, our mentors and our supporters were devastated. Many of the players were inconsolable and needed time to come to terms with the loss. I wasn't prepared for the result as I badly wanted us to win this title for Austin Stacks. I was satisfied, however, that the players had left everything on the field. They fought on like Corinthians to the bitter end. The team hadn't got the rub of the green on this occasion. It had been my policy during my entire term as Chairman that as a club we would win or lose together. We didn't practice the blame game and we would return home as a united club, broken but unbowed. The team had a lot to look forward to in the season ahead. I had no doubt that they were good enough and committed enough to be back in the Munster final again at the end of the season. If so, I would be supporting them from the terrace with much better sight. If the year went well my two corneal transplant operations and my second cataract surgery would have taken place. The success of those procedures now became my priority.

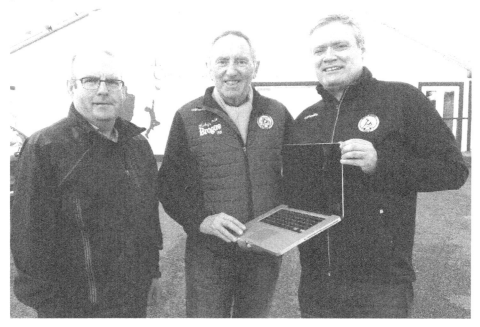

From left, Mike Tangney, Billy Ryle and Shane Lynch launch a fundraising drive, on the 11th January 2022, for the Munster Club Senior Football Final against St. Finbarrs of Cork.

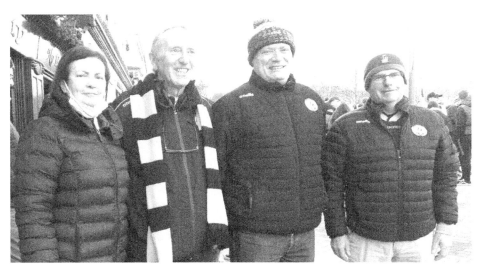

From left, Sheila & Billy Ryle, Shane Lynch and Mike Tangney were in Thurles on Sunday, 16th January 2022 for the Munster Club Senior Football Final

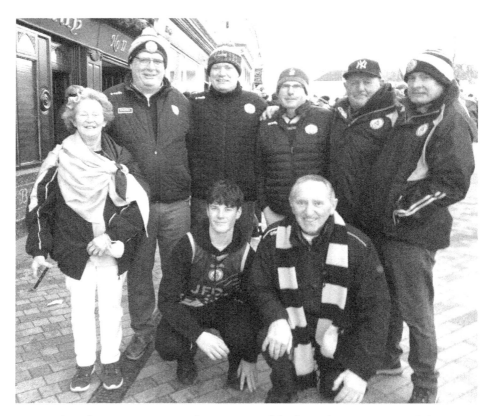

Austin Stacks supporters in happy mood before the Munster Club Senior Football Final in Thurles on Sunday, 16th January 2022. Front L/r Mark Lynch and Billy Ryle. Back L/r Carmel Quilter O'Neill, Liam & Shane Lynch, Mike Tangney, Jerry Carroll and David Prendergast

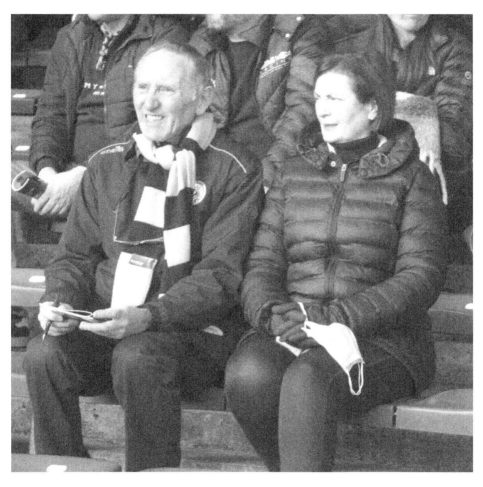

Tension is etched on the faces of Austin Stacks Club Chairman, Billy Ryle and his wife, Sheila as their team chases an equalising point in the Munster Club Senior Football Final in Semple Stadium, Thurles on Sunday, 16th January 2022

CHAPTER FORTY

STEPPING DOWN

During the days after the Thurles game, I availed of the opportunity to bring closure to my stewardship in a positive and encouraging manner. A number of media outlets had been in touch for a reaction to our defeat in the Munster final. I received the first phone call as my wife and I were a few kilometres outside Thurles on our journey home. I requested some time to gather my thoughts as I was still too emotional after the game to make any kind of objective comment. I promised to prepare a statement and issue it later on Sunday night.

I began by saying that as I was coming to terms with the loss of the game and the disappointment of elimination from the All-Ireland Senior Club Championship, my overriding emotion was one of immense pride in the team and the colourful supporters, who travelled to Thurles in huge numbers.

"Knocked back by the sucker punch of an early goal and being six points down at half-time, the lads turned in a superb second half to come within one point of St Finbarr's. Despite a great comeback our gallant side came up just short by 2-9 to 1-10 after playing their hearts out to the very end. Regardless of the loss in Thurles, our senior team has enjoyed wonderful success in 2021 – Kerry Senior Club Champions and Kerry Senior Football Champions. Congratulations to the team and mentors on a wonderful season and I'm very proud of each and every one of them," I added.

I expressed my sincere thanks to Austin Stacks supporters who made the journey in large numbers to Thurles and really got behind the team. "The atmosphere in the town square was electric and the parade to Semple Stadium was spectacular. The enthusiastic reception given by our supporters to our team after the final whistle brought a tear to my eye. Well done to the famous 16th Man," I said.

I congratulated St. Finbarr's and wished them good luck in the All-Ireland series. I also congratulated Na Gaeil, Gneeveguilla and Kilmoyley on their respective Munster title victories and hoped that they would go all the way to bring All-Ireland titles back to Kerry.

For the remainder of the week, I concentrated on the final preparations for our Annual General Meeting which would take place in our Club House in Connolly Park on Sunday, 23rd January 2022. There was a great turn out of members which pleased me as I regard the AGM as an ideal forum for open and honest debate. I opened the AGM with a few words of welcome.

"I'm delighted to welcome you to our AGM and I'm very pleased that so many members are present here this morning. Our AGM is a very important exercise in democracy, giving the leaders of the club an opportunity to account for their stewardship and giving you, the club members, a forum to express your views on club policy. No motions have been submitted, so I hope we'll have a very informative plenary session instead. What you have to say is important and your views and recommendations on any aspects of club policies are very welcome.

My sincere thanks to my colleagues on the Club Executive Committee, who provided solid, sensible and progressive leadership in 2021, which was a very special year with our victory in the Kerry Senior Football Championship, a century after the Rock Street Club won its first County Football Championship, at Junior level, in 1921.

As a new Chairman, Shane Lynch is taking office today I'd like to wish Shane every success in his leadership of Austin Stacks. I'm delighted that a younger member has stepped up to take the Chair. I sincerely hope that his example will be followed by more of his age group over the next few years. I'm always reluctant to give unsolicited advice, Shane. I know from working with you that you will be a very good Chairman but if you want to be a successful Chairman keep winning titles! The Rockies have an insatiable appetite for silverware!

Finally, I spoke with Club President, Brendan Dowling during the week. He asked me to convey his apologies and good wishes to today's AGM. He doesn't feel up to attending after the recent death of his lifelong friend, Ritchie McCarthy of Killeen and formerly Ballyduff. Ritchie won seven Senior County Hurling Championship medals with Ballyduff (1955-1965). He joined the Rock when he relocated to Tralee in the late sixties and was a member of a great Rock Hurling team that contested County Finals in 1968 and 1969 – two finals which we lost by the narrowest of margins. In addition to Ritchie and the great Jo Jo Barrett, The Rock lost some very fine people during the year. We fondly remember all of them today. I extend sincere sympathy to all members and supporters of Austin Stacks who suffered bereavement since our last AGM."

My opening remarks were followed by a comprehensive report from outgoing Club Secretary, Elma Nix. Club Treasurer, Mike Tangney was next up with a detailed financial report. It was reassuring to note that our finances were looking a great deal healthier than they were when I was elected Chairman in December 2019. My invitation to Shane Lynch and Mary Fitzmaurice to join the Club Executive as Assistant Treasures had proven very beneficial. Mike, Shane and Mary worked very effectively as a team and all three had an outstanding knowledge of financial management. As one who can just about micro manage my own financial affairs, I was very grateful for their prudent management of the Club's finances.

It was my turn text to present the Chairman's address. I told those present that 2021 had been a very successful year for The Rock both on and off the field. I said that we were all disappointed to lose the Munster Senior Club Football Final on the previous Sunday but it was worth remembering that in 2021 we had won our fair share of competitions up and down all ranks of the club.

"In particular, we won the County Senior Club Championship for the third year running as well as our first County Senior Football Championship since 2014. Our Senior B team won Division Five of the Senior County League and promotion to Division Four as well as winning the Junior League Division One in the Tralee and St Brendan's District. So, while we would all love to be preparing for the All-Ireland Senior Club Semi-Final, we can be very proud of the efforts of our team mentors and panels at all levels throughout the club," I added.

I made the point that winning trophies was very important, but it was equally gratifying to look back at the amount of activity that had been provided for players of all ages.

"That could not happen without the dedicated work of our coaches and I sincerely thank all of you for your service to Austin Stacks. From both administrative and playing perspectives, Austin Stacks is a well-organised and a well-structured club, with a tradition of winning competitions from juvenile to senior level. With our regular successes across all levels of the club, Austin Stacks will always be a major force in Kerry football," I emphasised.

"Effective up and down communication throughout our club was one of my key administrative objectives. It's vital for good management and high morale that all of us are fully informed about club policy and activities. Every member from Chairman to the newest member is entitled to information inclusion. So never assume in a club of this size that specific and general club activities are universally known. Get the information in circulation through word of mouth, our social media outlets and club notes. A well-informed membership makes a stronger club," I continued.

"The monthly meetings of our Club Executive Committee are business-like and productive. We share information. We have open and frank discussion and our decisions are democratically arrived at. Our deliberations are policy driven and our work is shared so that no member is overburdened. With that in mind, the subcommittees, which we set up during the last few years are very effective and have considerably enhanced the quality of service provided to our members. In addition to our existing subcommittees, namely JobMatch, Field, Lotto, Social, Finance, Juvenile, Gaeilge/Cultúir and Coaching/Games Development we have added Infrastructural Development and

Sponsorship. My thanks to all of you who have made yourselves available to serve on these subcommittees," I said.

"One of the administrative highlights for me this year was the production of the excellent coaching manual by our coaching committee, chaired by our excellent Vice-Chairman, Éamonn O'Reilly. This is a very valuable document which not only includes a detailed coaching platform but also the mission, vision and values of our Club. The chosen motto - TEAM – Together Everybody Achieves More – couldn't be more appropriate. We are all members of a club where the TEAM ethic is strong and that is why the club achieves so much at all levels.

Austin Stacks is very grateful to our sponsors for their generous financial support during a year where our successes resulted in considerable extra expenditure, namely - Kirby's Brogue Inn and Restaurant, our main sponsors from 2020 to 2023, Ned O'Shea & Sons Construction Ltd and John Lane & Sons Ltd, Food Service Distributors, who jointly sponsor Austin Stacks U-17, U-15 and U-13 football teams from 2021 to 2023, Ross Jewellers, sponsors of our U-11 teams in 2021 and Terry Healy of Terry's Butcher, sponsors of our Academy. My thanks also to John Murphy of Celsius Menswear, who sponsored our senior 'Man of the match' awards all year.

Through the O'Shea/Lane sponsorship we established a formal working relationship with Jigsaw Kerry, which is a free mental health service for young people. The jerseys of the O'Shea/Lane sponsored teams are displaying the logo, Jigsaw Kerry Youth Mental Health and Austin Stacks is availing of the expertise of Jigsaw Kerry to provide mental health information, support and counselling for our young players. I want to thank Mike Casey and Frank O'Rahilly for their great work in establishing this wonderful service," I said.

"All of us who are active in The Rock are doing so in a voluntary capacity. We do it for the great affection we have for Austin Stacks and for the personal satisfaction of contributing to a great club. Volunteers are rarely thanked and often criticised. I want to express my sincere gratitude to every member who has contributed to Austin Stacks in 2021 from our distinguished Club President, Brendan Dowling right through to our most humble and unassuming voluntary worker. One person who has given distinguished voluntary service to The Rock over many years as Club Secretary is Elma Nix, who is stepping down today after eight years in the position. On behalf of the entire club membership. I want to thank Elma for her dedicated work for Austin Stacks and also for her invaluable secretarial assistance to myself as Club Chairman.

It's been a great personal privilege to be Chairman of Austin Stacks and I hope that my time leading the Club has been productive both on and off the field. Under my Chairmanship, the club has undergone a root and branch review of its structures and many members have contributed to that process. Morale in The Rock is sky high due to the positive atmosphere permeating the club and to our outstanding success on the field. Further progress in these regards will be made by incoming Chairman, Shane Lynch, who is far more talented and youthful than myself. Shane, from Lisloose, has impeccable Austin Stacks pedigree, being the son of former Club Vice-Chairman, the late John Lynch and brother of former Chairman and current Vice-Chairman of Kerry County Board, Liam Lynch. I have given my heart, my soul and my energies to the Chairmanship during my term. I am delighted now to hand over the responsibility to a very safe pair of hands, a very gifted young man who will lead The Rock to further success," I said.

"I'd like to thank every club member for the courtesy shown to me and for your support and goodwill during my term in office. When I was elected Chairman of Austin Stacks, I took as my motto an adaptation of John Fitzgerald Kennedy's motto from his inauguration speech as President of the USA in January,1961. 'Ask not what your club can do for you. Rather ask what you can do for your club.' You responded with generosity during my tenure and I know you will continue to give and give again to this great club in the years ahead," I concluded.

The election of officers followed. I proposed Club President, Brendan Dowling for the position. Unfortunately, Brendan was called to his eternal reward during the year and the affable Aidan O'Connor was elected to the position of President at the AGM in January 2023.

Shane Lynch was then elected Chairman for the coming year, I congratulated Shane and wished him well for the year. Shane then took over as facilitator of the AGM and I took a seat in the general body of the meeting. I had mixed emotions. I would have liked to remain on as Chairman for a third and final year. But, in my heart, I knew that would not have been fair to the club nor to myself. The priority for the next twelve months had to be the correction of my vision. I was due to attend the Bon Secours Hospital in Cork in just four weeks for a corneal transplant of a donor organ in my right eye. In the build up to that surgery, I needed to avoid flu, Covid-19 and all other illnesses that might cause the operation to be deferred.

To bring down the curtain on my term as Chairman of Austin Stacks, I issued one final statement to our supporters through the club's media outlets. I had already explained to my colleagues on the Executive Committee why it was necessary for me to step aside as Chairman. I wasn't particularly keen to share my Fuchs Dystrophy with all and sundry so I didn't refer to it in my statement. Those who needed to know did know, so I left it at that.

In the statement which I released to the Club membership I said, "My term as Chairman of Austin Stacks GAA Club came to an end at a buoyant AGM at our club grounds in Connolly Park, Tralee last Sunday, 23rd January 2022. It's been a great personal privilege to have been Chairman of Austin Stacks and I hope that my time leading the Club has been productive both on and off the field. I'd like to sincerely thank the Club's Executive Committee, every club member and our loyal supporters for the courtesy shown to me and for your support and goodwill during my term in office.

Under my Chairmanship, the Club has undergone a root and branch review of its structures, a process to which many members have contributed. Morale in The Rock is sky high due to the positive atmosphere permeating the Club and to our outstanding success on the playing field. Further progress in these regards will be made by incoming Chairman, Shane Lynch, who is far more talented and youthful than myself. Shane, from Lisloose, Tralee has impeccable Austin Stacks pedigree, being the son of former Club Vice-Chairman, the late John Lynch and brother of former Chairman and current Vice-Chairman of Kerry County Board, Liam Lynch. I have given my heart, my soul and all of my energies to the Chairmanship during my term. I am delighted now to hand over the responsibility to a very safe pair of hands, a very gifted young man who will lead The Rock to further success both on and off the field."

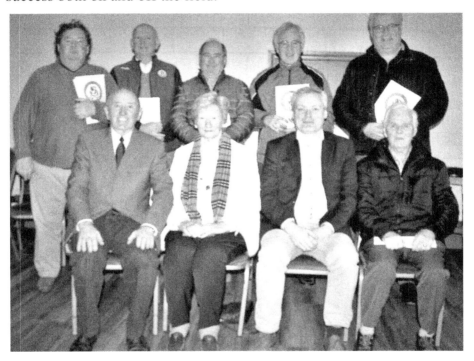

Former Chairpersons of Austin Stacks GAA Club, Tralee, pictured with incoming Chairman, Shane Lynch at the Club AGM on Sunday, 23rd January 2022 Front L/r: Billy Ryle, Mairéad Fernane, Shane Lynch and Tadhg McMahon Back L/r: Eddie Barrett, Jim Naughton, Michael Hickey, Aidan O'Connor and Liam Lynch

CHAPTER FORTY ONE

ANOTHER SETBACK

During the weeks before I was due in Cork for the surgery in my right eye, I took every precaution to remain fit and illness free. I swam in the sea on most days as sea swimming on an all-year-round basis has been my practice for many years. I really enjoyed the hour of exercise each day accompanied by my faithful dog, Jake. I practiced social distancing, wore a protective mask in crowded situations and did my best to avoid colds and flues and of course the omnipresent Covid–19. I was in great shape for an operation – if that doesn't sound contradictory – when another setback confronted me. Word came from Cork that my corneal transplant surgery which was scheduled for Thursday, 10th February 2022 would have to be postponed to a later date. This news was very disappointing as I was certain that the operation would go ahead this time without a hitch. As the song says, "my bags are packet and I'm ready to go," except I no longer had a place to which I could go. There had been a ten-week gap between the first and second postponements so I expected that it would be another two or three months before I would be given a new date for the corneal transplant surgery.

I did my best to remain positive and continued with best practice in my life style in order to be fit and ready for the call for the rescheduled operation. I reread the information I had about Fuchs Dystrophy to reassure myself that I understood, as much as a layman could, what the disease was and that I fully comprehended the seriousness of undergoing an operation that would transplant an organ from a donor into my eye. The fact that the operation had been postponed twice made me realise that the procedure was far more than a routine surgery. My self-confidence was beginning to be knocked back and I was again faced with a few psychological issues which I had earlier resolved. Should I have left things as they were? Would my vision stabilise without any further deterioration? Would I be worse off if things went wrong? What if I finish up blind? All of these questions were crossing my mind and I was beginning to run a little bit scared. I was forced to have a few serious chats with myself.

Mr Flynn had gone through all the issues with me. I had been anxious to have the corrective procedures from the start. I was determined from the outset to meet the Fuchs headlong and to do everything in my power to maintain my vision at a functional level which would allow me to live an independent life. I reminded myself of the recent game in Thurles when I was looking at a hazy pitch. No, I'm not expressing that correctly. I was looking with blurred vision at a perfect pitch because of the deterioration in my eye sight. If I backed out now, I'd very likely spent my days on the couch listening to the broadcast of football matches rather than watching them from the terrace. What if I could never read another book? As an inveterate reader, I'd be devastated without the great joy of picking up a good book. My daily trip to Fenit with Jake for a stroll and an invigorating dip in the sea would be at an end. I needed to pull myself together. I had nothing to fear but fear itself. I had full confidence in Mr Flynn. I needed to have confidence in myself.

To keep myself motivated I looked at the definition of Fuchs Dystrophy. It's a build-up of fluid in the cornea on the front of the eye, which causes blurred vision. When the Fuchs has advanced to a stage where a person's vision is affecting the person's ability to function well, corneal transplant surgery of a donor organ is the best way to improve vision. The prognosis for a person with severe Fuchs Dystrophy who doesn't have the transplant is not good. Severe pain, reduced vision and even blindness are consequences of inaction.

That decided it for me. I would proceed according to plan and meet the Fuchs Dystrophy headlong. I had to be brave and resilient. I am often called 'the delivery man' because of my ability to get things done whether in family life, in sport or education. Now I had to press ahead and deliver for myself. All my doubts and introspection came to an abrupt end when a letter arrived informing me to report to the Admissions Department, Bon Secours Hospital, College Road, Cork at

12.30pm on the 7th of April 2022 for corneal transplant surgery in my right eye. I was delighted with the news and immediately set about collecting my eye drops from the Pharmacist, organising my overnight bag and arranging my transport to Cork. I said a silent prayer to St. Martin De Porres, the Black Friar of Lima, Peru, my Patron Saint, that it would be a case of third time lucky and that all would go well. I was prepared to cross my Rubicon and not look back in anger! Rather, like Caesar, I would march forward with resilience.

CHAPTER FORTY TWO

FIRST CORNEAL TRANSPLANT

I travelled by 9am train from Tralee to Cork on Thursday, 7th April 2022. I don't recall a great deal about the journey other than the fact that the seats around me were vacant. I glossed over the headlines in the daily paper but I didn't have the concentration nor the vision to read the articles in detail. I closed my eyes but sleep wouldn't come so most of my journey was spent either looking out the window or waiting for the next stop for passengers to get on board or to disembark. Farranfore, Killarney, Rathmore, Millstreet and Banteer were serviced and the train soon arrived at Mallow which was the terminus for this train. The platform was crowded with people waiting for connecting trains to come and go. The Cork train to Dublin pulled in and passengers heading for the capital got on board. My impatience grew is I waited for the Dublin to Cork train to pull in. On previous occasions the train had been a few minutes late in arriving into Mallow. I was hoping that it would arrive on time as I waited with the people heading into Cork. Some were going shopping. Others were heading for college lectures. Some were keeping medical appointments of one sort or another. I was heading for surgery that very afternoon. As I stood on the platform, with my journey at a standstill, I began to think of the late individual whose cornea would be implanted into my right eye in a few hours. How had that person died? Was the donor male or female? Would I ever know who the person was? Unlikely, I thought, as organ donors remain anonymous to the best of my knowledge.

The shrill sound from the whistle of the approaching train stirred me from my melancholic reflections. I jumped on the train which moved off without delay as soon as all the Cork bound passengers had boarded. About thirty minutes later the train arrived at Kent Station, Cork. It was approaching noon so I headed for the taxi rank, where there was a line of expectant drivers awaiting the arrival of the Dublin train. I hopped into the back of the next taxi in line and I informed the driver of my destination.

"Are you visiting someone or are you going under the knife, like?" inquired the taxi driver in an accent which left me in no doubt that he was a native Corkonian.

"They wouldn't even allow Roy Keane inside the door of the Bons at present unless he was a patient because of the strict visiting restrictions," I replied, in an attempt to deflect the conversation away from myself.

The digression worked as the driver responded in the manner in which I was hoping he would.

"Aarragh boy, Roy could talk his way into Heaven, like. Sure, he's better than any of the British fellas on the BBC during the soccer matches."

To the best of my knowledge, Roy was a soccer analyst with ITV but as I was beginning to enjoy the banter, I continued to keep the conversation going.

"Roy would have made the Cork senior football team if he hadn't taken up the soccer," I quipped.

"Naw, they're hopeless and he'd have made no money. He's a lot better off where he is and he gets in free to all the games, boy."

Sometime late as we travelled up College Road after a nice distracting chat about Roy and the affection that Cork people had for him, he said, "Here we are now. I'll drive you up to the entrance because I see a few drops of rain on the windscreen."

"You're a gentleman and what's the damage?" I inquired.

"€15 to you, boy. I handed him €20 and told him to keep the change.

"Thanks very much and I hope you'll be alright, boy."

He had spotted my overnight bag as I got out of the car. I appreciated the comment even if you can't beat The Rebels for roguery.

The Covid -19 protocols at the Hospital, as you'd expect, were very tight. I donned my facemask and sanitized my hands at the entrance lobby which had a very conspicuous "NO VISITORS ALLOWED" sign placed on the facing wall. Having satisfied the security guard with the knowledge that I was signing-in as a patient, I was directed to the Admissions Department, where I was told to take a seat and I would be admitted in due course. It was 12.20pm. My call came at 12.40pm and I was directed to a booth where I was asked a lot of questions about my personal details and my medical history. The administrator also confirmed all the details of the procedure for which I was been admitted. I signed the form of confirmation and was escorted to the pre-operation ward where I sat by the bed. I was given a preliminary examination by a member of the nursing staff and an outline of the surgery ahead of me. A house Doctor arrived sometime later and checked my details and took me, once again through the details on my operation. She asked me to confirm which eye was for surgery. I had to think for a moment as the strange surroundings had thrown me slightly off-guard.

"It's the right eye, I think. Yes, definitely, it's the right eye," I replied.

"Right eye and right answer," she laughed.

Another nurse came in some time later and once again took my blood pressure and did some other pre-operative procedures. She said that she was a member of the Theatre Staff and would be with me during the operation. She told me to remove my upper clothes and shoes and to change into the gown that was by my bed. I then sat into the trolly bed where the back was upright. I was told that I would be wheeled to the operating theatre where I would be given a local anaesthetic and the transplant would then be performed by Mr Flynn. I remember being rolled up to the operating theatre where I was put lying in a horizontal position in preparation for the procedure. An Anaesthetist explained how the anaesthetic would be administered and how it would numb the area around the eye. Any discomfort during the operation would be minimal he told me. Mr Flynn had earlier called to the pre-operative room to put a pencil mark over my right eye. The Anaesthetist still asked me to confirm which eye was for surgery. I appreciated their thoroughness.

It was a strange experience to be awake for the operation. My entire face was covered by a sterile strip except for the right eye. I could hear the dialogue going on all around me but, to me it seemed as if they were talking about someone else as I was hidden by the facial cover and I had no feeling in the right eye. I settled into my position and tried my best not to move my head as I had been instructed beforehand to remain as still as possible during the surgery. I began to appreciate what was happening all around me. This was what I had been waiting for and now I was begin operated on by Mr Flynn, who was one of the best in his field of expertise. The calmness and the efficiency of the medical team was very reassuring. Mr Flynn told me from time to time that all was going well. I was visualising each step in my head. The damaged cornea would be removed. Then the donor organ would be put in place. I knew it wasn't as simple as that and things could go wrong at any stage. I lost track of time and had no idea how close the operation was to a conclusion when Mr Flynn told me that the transplant had gone well. A bandage would be placed over the eye and I should lie still for some time before being returned to the pre-operation room. I must have dozed off until I heard somebody telling me that I was being returned to the room I had come from. I remained there for about an hour under supervision until Mr Flynn came in to examine the eye. He was very pleased with the outcome and bandaged the eye. A clear plastic shield was then placed over the eye and I was instructed to wear the shield at night for the first four days after the transplant surgery to help prevent inadvertent injury to the eye during sleep.

Sometime later I was transferred to a patient's room and requested to lie on my back during the night. I was mentally exhausted after the experience and only awoke when the night nurse came into the room to check on me. I recall a lady arriving into the room early the following morning to ask what I would like for breakfast. Only then did I realise that I was hungry and I ordered porridge, toast and tea to celebrate the arrival of a new day with a new cornea in my right eye.

CHAPTER FORTY THREE

AFTERCARE OF NEW CORNEA

On the evening of my corneal transplant surgery, I just about managed to send a text to my wife letting her know that I was back resting in a patient's room and that I expected to be discharged the following day. Mr Flynn had given me an early appointment for the following morning and, all being well, I could go home afterwards. Sheila was driving to Cork to collect me as the Hospital had a strict policy of only discharging a patient into the care of a responsible adult. Printing the text took some effort as my right eye was covered and the vision in my left eye was fuzzy.

After breakfast, I was escorted downstairs to meet with Mr Flynn at his clinic in the Bon Secours Hospital. He gave the right eye a thorough examination and seemed to be pleased with the outcome of the surgery. He told me that the transplant would take a few days to settle and he would see me at The Elysian early the following week. I was escorted back to my room where I dressed and prepared to leave for home. My wife had arrived but was not allowed to join me in my room due to the no visiting policy which was in force. I appreciated that was a necessary precaution and in turn I was escorted down to the front entrance where I was formally handed over to the care of my wife. My final task was to sign out at the Admissions Department. We had planned to have lunch but as I was still a bit flaky after the operation, we headed directly home where I rested for the remainder of the day.

For the first few weeks after the surgery, I was putting antibiotic drops and anti-inflammatory drops into my right eye. In order to be certain of using the appropriate drop at the right time, I made out a timetable for each type of drop. I found this very helpful as I was able to place a tick after each drop when I had placed it in my eye. I did forget from time to time, but overall, I was diligent in meeting the schedule. My eye remained covered for a few days and I wore the plastic shield in bed for four consecutive nights. I knew that I would have to take things easy for the first week after the procedure. That was not going to be a problem as I had accomplished it comfortably after the cataract surgery. Not being able to swim in the sea for four weeks after the surgery was another matter altogether, especially as the summer swimming season was getting underway. As one who is addicted to sea swimming, I missed the daily dip. Still, it was for my own good and my dog, Jake and I were still able to enjoy our daily stroll from the carpark in Fenit back to the bathing slip and watch the swimmers treading water. I wasn't driving myself at this early stage but I had no shortage of offers of lifts from my swimming buddies.

I travelled to Cork by 9am train from Tralee on Wednesday, 13th April 2022 for my first post-operative appointment with Mr Flynn. It was now six days since the transplant had taken place. Vision in the right eye was getting better with each passing day. I was delighted that the haziness was completely gone and I could see better than I had for some time. There was some redness in the eye but I was aware from Mr Flynn's notes that it would clear after a few days. I walked from Kent Station, Cork to The Elysian in Eglinton St as the day was dry and pleasant. After an initial testing of my vision by Eanna, the Optician, my right eye was given a detailed examination by Mr Flynn. He was very pleased that the donor organ had settled very satisfactorily into my right eye. He told me to expect a gradual improvement in my vision and that all was well.

I was back again on the following week. My appointment was fixed for 12pm on Tuesday, 19th April 2022. It was now twelve days after the right eye corneal transplantation. Mr Flynn told me that the cornea oedema had improved further since the previous week's visit and the visual acuity had already improved to the best level it had been in years. Everything I heard from Mr Flynn was music to my ears. He had played his part and I was determined to continue to remain disciplined in my drop taking, in my compliance with social distancing and in my avoidance of situations where I might be at risk of infection. Mr Flynn said he would see me in about three weeks.

My next appointment was fixed for 12pm on Tuesday, 10th May 2022. It was now about five weeks after my surgery. Mr Flynn told me that the eye had settled very well and that my vision had continued to improve in the period since I had received the organ transplant. He removed the stitches from my eye and said I could make an appointment in Tralee with Dr O'Regan for new glasses. That was great news. The spectacles would benefit my right eye only as the haze in my left eye would only be eliminated by cataract surgery followed by corneal transplantation. In other words, the two procedures which Mr Flynn had carried out on my right eye would now need to be repeated on my left eye. Mr Flynn said he would see me in about eight weeks and we would discuss left eye surgery at that stage. I was half way in the journey to improve my sight. It had taken much longer that I had expected from the time I was first diagnosed with Fuchs Dystrophy in January 2018. My next appointment with Mr Flynn was fixed for 12.30pm on Wednesday, 29th June 2022. At that stage, half of 2022 would have passed. I wondered what the next half year held in store for me.

CHAPTER FORTY FOUR

CATARACT & CORNEA

A few days after my appointment with Mr Flynn, I attended the First Holy Communion of my eldest grandchild, Kate Ryle at the Church of the Purification, Churchill, Tralee on Saturday, 14th May 2022. It was a wonderful day of celebration for the Ryle and Higgins families as Kate was the first of the new generation of the Ryle family to receive the Sacrament. There was a lovely atmosphere in the Church and it brought back many happy memories of my own children receiving the Sacraments. Our group enjoyed a relaxing meal afterwards at the local Oyster Tavern Restaurant in Spa Village.

The following evening, on Sunday, 15th May 2022, Sheila and I attended a documentary on the life of St. Brendan, the Patron Saint of Kerry at the Rose Hotel in Tralee. I have had a great interest in St. Brendan since I was a boy as he was born in Fenit where I swim regularly. I was also a member of the fundraising committee which was responsible for the building of the magnificent monument of St Brendan which was blessed and unveiled by The Bishop of Kerry, Bill Murphy on Sunday, 19th September 2004. The monument dominates Tralee Bay from its lofty position on Samphire Rock. Another reason for our attendance at the launch of the documentary was that it was produced by Éamonn O'Reilly, my trusted Vice-Chairman of Austin Stacks. Is there no limit to this man's talents?

On Tuesday, 7th June, 2022, I had an appointment in Tralee with Dr Tom O'Regan, Consultant Ophthalmologist. Dr O'Regan was delighted that the corneal transplant had been so successful and he measured my eyes for updated glasses. He suggested that I use two pairs for the moment, one pair for reading and the second for distance. I couldn't belief the improvement in my vision when I tried on the new glasses a few days later. I was able to read the daily paper, standard font books and all other documentation with no difficulty at all. It was wonderful. It had been a few years since I had enjoyed this comfort level of reading. It had always been a concern to me that my capacity to read standard material might not be restored. I am a passionate reader and the loss of my ability to pursue one of my favourite hobbies would have left a huge void in my life.

The distance glasses change my life completely. Even though I hadn't done any long-distance driving since I was diagnosed with Fuchs Dystrophy, I was well able to cover short distances. It gave me great independence. Most of all, I was now able to return to watching football games. I hadn't been at an Austin Stacks game since the Munster Senior Club Football Final in Thurles the previous January, but now I had much greater clarity in my right eye. My enjoyment of the games was considerably enhanced and I was able to read the electronic scoreboard on the far side of the pitch for the first time in ages. I travelled to the away games with my friends Mairéad and Tim and even if the results were not as good as they had been when I was Chairman, I was thrilled to be there to support our teams. I'm around long enough to know that both success and failure are transient occurrences. They come and go like the seasons. The mark of any good club is to remain steadfast in good times and bad. I have constantly stated that we will always stand and fall together. Most of all, we will get up off of the ground together, dust ourselves down and start winning matches as a united club. The blame game has no place in our philosophy.

As no glasses could make any improvement to the vision in my left eye, Dr O Regan said he would provide me with a long-term pair of glasses when that second eye had been operated on. I was looking forward to that day but there was further surgery to be done first.

A few weeks later, on Wednesday, 29th June, I returned to Cork for my appointment with Mister Flynn. After a thorough examination of my eyes by Mr Flynn, he informed me that the corneal graft in my right eye was functioning well and he was very pleased with my considerably improved vision. He told me that the vision in my left eye had considerably reduced due to a combination of cataract and corneal oedema. He added that cataract surgery is normally done first and that corneal transplantation follows sometime later if it's required. In my case, as I was suffering from Fuchs Dystrophy, both cataract and corneal transplant surgery were required. We discussed the risks and benefits of combined cataract surgery with corneal endothelial transplantation. The main benefit was the good chance of improving vision. The risks were

1) A 10% chance of graft dislocation requiring further surgery
2) Glaucoma
3) Graft failure
4) A one in five hundred chance of a loss of vision from intraocular infection

I was keen to proceed with the combined surgery and Mr Flynn was happy to perform it, so we agreed to go ahead with the surgery. Mr Flynn told me he would need to perform a preoperative laser peripheral iridotomy in the left eye in the Outpatients' Department at Bons Secours Hospital, Cork. Laser peripheral iridotomy uses laser energy to create a small hole in the Iris, the coloured part at the front of the eye, to help open the drainage angle. The procedure takes about ten minutes and the hole is not visible to the naked eye. Mr Flynn said he would arrange a date for the laser procedure and he would then schedule a date for the combined surgery. He told me to continue with the eyedrops in accordance with the prescription. Sometime after that appointment, I received correspondence informing me that an appointment had been arranged for my procedure with Mr Flynn at 10am on Thursday, 22nd September 2022 at the Outpatients' Department, Bon Secours Hospital, College Road, Cork.

CHAPTER FORTY FIVE

ENJOYING THE GAMES

I enjoyed attending the Austin Stacks football matches during August and September. The club was defending both the Senior Club Championship and the County Senior Football Championship. Up first was the Senior Club Championship where we were drawn in Group Two with Templenoe, Kerins O'Rahillys and Dr Crokes. Surprisingly, we suffered a fairly heavy defeat to Templenoe in our first group game. The game, which was played in Derreen, Killarney on Sunday, 7th August 2022 finished on a scoreline of 2-12 to 1-8. A week later on a very warm Sunday afternoon, 14th August 2022, in Connolly Park, we just got over the line for a very valuable victory against a game Kerins O'Rahillys side by 1-15 to 1-14.

We travelled to play Dr Crokes in Killarney on Sunday, 21st August 2022 for a game that both sides needed to win. This was our third and final Group Two game in the senior club championship. Unfortunately, things didn't go Austin Stacks way and we suffered a five-point defeat on a score of 1-13 to 0-11. Our Senior Club title was now gone and we were left facing a relegation play-off against Kenmare Shamrocks, who finished fourth in Group One. That game would determine which of the two teams would be relegated to Intermediate status for the following year.

A successful defence of our County Senior Football title now became the focus of our attention. On a pleasant Friday evening, 9th September 2022 at Austin Stack Park we began the defence of our title against local rivals Na Gaeil. It was a keenly contested game where we always had a very slight edge. Final score was Austin Stacks 0-14 Na Gaeil 1-8. Our second game in Group Three was at home against West Kerry on Saturday evening, 17th September. On an ideal evening for football, we notched up an impressive win against a disappointing West Kerry side by 2-13 to 1-8 to qualify for the quarter-finals of the County Senior Football Championship.

Our senior team travelled to Beaufort on Sunday afternoon, 25th September 2002 to play Mid Kerry in the third and final game of our group. Both teams had already qualified for the last eight so the game was all about topping the group. It was virtually certain that hot favourites East Kerry, with David and Paudie Clifford on board, would top their Group. The winning team in Beaufort would be in the same bowel as East Kerry and the losing team would be in the runners-up bowel. A win could be important depending on how the quarter-final draws turned out. Austin Stacks never got going in this game and lost heavily by 1-15 to 1-7. Despite the defeat, the quarter-final draw was very kind to The Rock when we were pitted against Feale Rangers at Austin Stack Park. It was almost as good as a home draw and our supporters were expected to turn out in large numbers.

We were hopeful if not our usual confident selves as we gathered in Austin Stack Park on Saturday, 8th October 2022 for our Senior Football Championship quarter final game with Feale Rangers, who got off to a great start with two early points. However, for the remainder of the half they only added a single point to five points for Austin Stacks. We were happy at the interval break. In a closely contested second half Feale Rangers outscored us by six points to four to tie the game nine points each at full time. The tension was unbearable as it was all to play for. Unfortunately, we failed to score in the first period of extra time while our opponents added a goal and a point. Austin Stacks did outscore Feale Rangers by three points to two in the second period of extra time but the damage had been done in the first period of extra time. Austin Stacks surrendered the Kerry Senior Football Championship title by 1-12 to 0-12. Feale Rangers advanced to the semi-finals of the competition.

After poor performances in both the Senior Club Championship and the Senior County Championship, Austin Stacks was now under severe pressure to retain its senior status. We had beaten Kenmare Shamrocks in the final of the Senior Club Championship in 2020 and 2021. Now we needed to beat them again or Austin Stacks would be playing

Intermediate football for the first time in its history. The game was fixed for Fitzgerald Stadium on Sunday 23rd October, 2022. The Rockie supporters travelled in numbers to support their team. They knew what was at stake. A defeat was incomprehensible.

Its often said that goals win games and that was the case in this relegation game in Killarney. Kenmare rattled the net three times to build up a big lead of 3-2 to 0-4. Our team replied in style and had the gap reduced to three points at the interval break, Kenmare Shamrocks 3-5 Austin Stacks 1-8. At that stage, I felt we had weathered the storm.

For some unknown reason, we scored only a single point in the third quarter and found ourselves behind by 3-10 to 1-9 with about ten minutes to go. Although we finished strongly with a further six points to a single point by our opponents, we had left ourselves with too much too do. Austin Stacks was relegated to Intermediate status on a final score line of 3-11 to 1-15.

It was a year on the field which we won't remember with any great fondness. As well as suffering relegation from Senior status, our Senior B team was relegated from the County League Division Four to Division Five. It was a pity because our Senior B squad had gone undefeated in Divisional Five in 2021 to win promotion and had won the Division Five Final to boot. But 2023 is another year. Hopefully, Austin Stacks will get the rub of the green and our players will not be side-lined by the injuries that plagued the team in 2022. Austin Stacks belongs in the Kerry Senior Football Championship. I am confident that The Rock will once again be playing senior football in 2024.

CHAPTER FORTY SIX

COMBINED SURGERY

Sheila and I travelled to Cork by car on the 22nd September 2022 for the outpatient procedure at the Bon Secours Hospital. Mr Flynn performed the laser peripheral iridotomy on my left eye. The procedure was an uncomplicated surgery which was over in about fifteen minutes and I was allowed to leave shortly afterwards. Sheila and I headed down to the Wilton Restaurant where we enjoyed breakfast and after some shopping at the Wilton Shopping Centre we drove home. I was back in Cork the following Tuesday, 27th September for an appointment with Mr Flynn at The Elysian. After an examination of my left eye, Mr Flynn was happy that all appeared well following my laser iridotomy procedure of the previous week. He said that he would proceed with the combined cataract surgery and corneal endothelial transplant. Shortly after that visit I received correspondence informing me of the admission details for my surgery with Mr Flynn. I was to report to the Admissions Department, Bon Secours Hospital, College Road Cork at 12.30pm on Thursday, 10th November 2022. As was the case with my right eye corneal transplant, I would have to stay in Hospital overnight.

A few days before I was due to travel to Cork, I noticed a small red bump on the lower lid of my right eye. The official name for the red bump is a chalazion. I did not know that at the time and I expected it would clear itself. When I met with Mr Flynn at the Hospital on the day of the surgery, he was very concerned about the chalazion. Even though he was going to operate on my left eye, he was concerned that the chalazion under my right eye might cause some cross-infection. The donor organ was ready to be transplanted but I realised that Mr Flynn had some reservations about going ahead with the procedures because of this unforeseen risk presented by the chalazion. As I felt a bit guilty about wasting a suitable organ, I told him that I'd be happy to go ahead with the operation if he felt it was safe to do so.

Mr Flynn said he would come back to me in a little while with a decision. He later told me that he had contacted a number of his fellow Consultant Ophthalmic Surgeons for their opinions. I was very impressed and, indeed, very grateful that a man with his medical expertise in corneal transplantation would go to the trouble of double checking with his colleagues. I was confident that whatever decision he made would be made in the best interests of the patient, who in this instance was myself. When Mr Flynn returned, he said that both he and his colleagues felt it would be safe to proceed with the surgery. I was very pleased about that because I was all psyched up and ready to go.

Just as was the case for the right eye corneal transplant, the preparation for the operation was thorough and diligent. It may have been my imagination, but I felt that everybody in the operation theatre was aware of the fact that this was a combined procedure which carrier an added risk due to the chalazion. I vaguely recall the Anaesthetist asking me if I was a keen exercise enthusiast as he looked at my medical chart before he anaesthetised the area of the eye.
"I'm a keen sea swimmer," I replied, "How did you know?"
"All your impressive medical readings give the tale away" he laughed.

That interaction gave me a timely boost. As he raised the syringe to administer the jab, a line from Macbeth's famous soliloquy crossed my mind– "is this a dagger which I see before me?" So, to make assurance doubly sure, I made one of my many intercessions to St Martin de Porres. I know that I torment the poor man, but he never lets me down. Now, I was once again asking him for another favour.

I have no idea how long the combined procedure lasted as I tried to remain as stable as possible for the duration. As I picked up bits and pieces of the dialogue between Mr Flynn and the theatre staff, I got the impression that all was going well. The fact that I was having cataract surgery as well as corneal transplantation suggested that I would be on the operating theatre for a longer period than was the case for the right eye corneal transplantation. Every step of the combined procedure was done calmly and with great precision. Eventually, I heard Mr Flynn saying that it was all over in an upbeat voice that portrayed satisfaction with a job well done. He then added "let's clean up the right eye." I recall feeling some eyedrops followed by the eye being covered with ointment. It felt good.

The left eye was bandaged and I was left on the trolly bed for some time before being rolled back to the pre-operation ward where I slept for a while. I remember Mr Flynn arriving to examine my eyes and telling me that the entire procedure had been very successful. A clear plastic eye shield was placed over the eye and I was transferred to a hospital room where I was to spend the night. Before I settled down for the night, I just about managed to send a text message to my wife to let her know that all had gone well and that I would see her on the following day. My left eye was bandaged and my right eye was sticky from the ointment but I was the happiest man in Cork city that night.

After an early breakfast the following morning, I was escorted down to my morning after appointment with Mr Flynn. After examining both eyes, he confirmed that the combined procedure had gone very well but the next few weeks would be critical. He had already prescribed antibiotic eyedrops and anti-inflammatory eyedrops for my left eye. He also prescribed strong antibiotic tablets and ointment for the chalazion in the right eye. I knew I would have to make out a schedule when I returned home. This time I'd have to be very vigilant as I was now on drops for both eyes in addition to the tablet and the ointment for the right eye. Once again, I prepared a timetable for the medications, which proved to be very helpful. My wife Sheila was also a great help with her regular reminders. "Don't forget your eyedrop" or "I hope you've taken your tablet" or "It's time to apply the ointment" were regular retorts sent in my direction. I'd be a bit annoyed with myself if I'd slipped up along the way, but I'd never admit it. "On the ball with everything," I'd reply and when the coast was clear, I'd get back on schedule. Sheila's promptings were invaluable during those early weeks when I was top heavy with medication and she knew well that I appreciated her support.

I was extremely careful in the weeks immediately following the surgery. I complied fully with the post-operative instruction provided in Mr Flynn's literature. It was difficult but necessary. The vision in my left eye started to return after a few days and continued to improve.

CHAPTER FORTY SEVEN

CHALAZION

I was back on the train again on Tuesday, 15th November 2022 on my way to Cork for an appointment with Mr Flynn at the Elysian. Eanna, the Optician checked my vision and then Mr Flynn did a detailed examination of both eyes. He said that the corneal transplant looked very well and the swelling in the chalazion had reduced. I still had some discomfort on the lower lid of the right eye but it had not interfered with the successful transplant in the left eye. Mr Flynn asked me to continue applying the eyedrops as prescribed and to return in a fortnight's time. I was given an appointment for 12.20pm on Tuesday, 29th November 2022.

I was beginning to get a bit curious about this chalazion so I took it upon myself to do a little bit of research. I wanted to learn what exactly a chalazion was. From my research I learned that a chalazion is a red bump on your eyelid. It is sometimes called an eyelid cyst or a meibomian cyst. It slowly forms when an oil gland, called a meibomian, becomes blocked. At first, the chalazion may be painful, but after a little time, it usually doesn't hurt.

What causes the red bump? Several oil glands in the eyelids secrete oils to moisten and protect your eyes. The glands can block and swell into a hard lump, known as a chalazion, if these oils become thick and waxy. Sometimes the hard lump can flare up and get infected, causing pain and redness.

How long should a chalazion last? In most cases the chalazion requires minimal medical treatment and clears up on its own in a few weeks to a month.

What happens if a chalazion is left untreated? Although it is an annoyance to most who periodically get a chalazion, it is not inherently dangerous or does not cause serious vision issues. If left untreated however, it can become more than a mere aggravation and eventually a chalazion can result in more serious visual issues.

Is a chalazion serious? In most cases a chalazion causes no problems. Rarely, a cyst can become infected and this infection can spread to involve the whole eyelid and tissues surrounding the eye. The eyelid may be very swollen and red. You might not be able to open the eye and you may have a lot of pain and a high temperature.

What cream removes chalazion? Patients are prescribed chloramphenicol ointment four times per day for five days, with gentle massage for five minutes after each ointment application. They are then followed up in three weeks. If the chalazion recurs, additional injections may be required.

How do you get rid of a chalazion? Your Ophthalmologist begins by administering a local anesthetic to numb the area around the cyst. The doctor then places a clamp on your eyelid to hold it still during the chalazion excision procedure. After making a tiny incision at the chalazion, the eye doctor uses a specialized instrument to remove the cyst.

The information was very informative and it was reassuring to learn that the chalazion wasn't directly linked to the cornea transplant. I had to remain vigilant in cleaning my eyes and to take care not to rub them. If the ointment and the antibiotic hadn't fully cleared the chalazion, I intended to discuss it with Mr Flynn at my next appointment on the 11th January 2003. By the time that appointment came around, it would be five years since Mr Wallace had first diagnosed my Fuchs Dystrophy. It had been a tough battle since then but, thank God, I had survived it and had been lucky with the successful surgeries.

I noticed that the letter informing me of this next appointment also contained advice regarding Covid-19 safety measures. Both the Bon Secours Hospital, Cork and Mr Flynn's Eye Clinic at The Elysian, Eglinton St, Cork insisted on a very high standard of safety measures so I hoped that the country was not facing another wave of the coronavirus pandemic. As requested, I carefully read the advice contained in the letter.

Patients were advised to contact the Eye Clinic and not attend for appointment if

1. You have symptoms of Covid-19
2. You have been in contact with someone who has tested positive for Covid-19
3. You have recently travelled to/from an affected region in the past 14 days

The following symptoms of Covid-19 were contained in the letter

1. A fever: high temperature – 38 degrees Celsius or above
2. A cough: this can be any kind of cough, not just dry
3. Shortness of breath or breathing difficulties

When attending for appointment, patients were requested to bring a facemask and wear it during the appointment

1. Use hand gel provided on entering and leaving your appointment
2. Only attend the appointment at the time given and not before
3. If you are over the age of eighteen and do not require a special assistant, please attend the appointment alone. If the patient is under the age of eighteen one parent should attend only. If the patient does require special assistance, one person, also wearing a facemask, should only come with the patient.
4. Check in at the reception desk in Mr Tom Flynn's office and the Secretary will instruct you on where to wait.
5. Please ensure to bring a mobile phone with you for your appointment in case you are required to wait in your car/elsewhere until called.

I fully appreciated that the measures outlined above were necessary for the patient's safety, the safety of the staff and everyone entering the Eye Clinic at The Elysian. Indeed, as a patient who had undergone two corneal transplants, I was very conscious of the risks of infection, inflammation and even rejection. I for one, was determined to remain as fully compliant with the safety measures as I had been from the outset.

CHAPTER FORTY EIGHT

THE CHARGE TO THE SEA

As I mention earlier, I have been an enthusiastic participant in the Christmas Day swim at noon in Fenit for longer that I care to remember. There is something magical about lining up on the beach with the huge crowd of participants and joining in the rendition of Jingle Bells at five minutes to mid-day. Then counting down from ten second to noon and charging headlong into the freezing sea. It's a long-standing tradition and whets the appetite for dinner. After my cataract surgery on the 18th December 2019, I didn't line up with the multitude of swimmers for the charge into the sea. I remained one step removed from the crowd and calmy strolled into the sea up to knee deep in the water. It really tested my willpower not to dive headlong into the sea but I accepted that it could not happen on this occasion. I had been given clear instructions by Mister Flynn which I was determined to follow. It wasn't the best Christmas swim I've ever had, but I did participate by stepping into the water and I really enjoyed the craic and the atmosphere that is unique to Fenit on Christmas.

Covid-19 put paid to the public Christmas Day swim in Fenit both in 2020 and 2021 so I was looking forward to the swim on Christmas Day 2022. On Christmas Day in 2020 and 2021, instead of charging to the ocean in the midst of the madding crowd, I enjoyed a relaxed early afternoon dip at the bathing slip in Fenit to whet the appetite for the Christmas dinner and to maintain my tradition of a Christmas plunge. It was lovely to see people taking a stroll or a dip while observing social distancing. I was pleased that all concerned were observing the NPHET protocols.

 The swims in 2020 and 2021 were akin to a spiritual experience, reminding me of the fragility of life and nature. I had always taken the swim for granted as part of my Christmas day routine. However, the pandemic had taught me to ground myself in the moment and live each day to the full within the restrictions that applied at the time. As one accustomed to swimming in choppy waters, I dedicated my Christmas dips in 2020 and 2021 to Dr Tony Holohan, a selfless national hero, who swam against a very strong tide to lead us safely through the difficult years of the coronavirus pandemic.

Indeed, the annual Christmas Day swim in Fenit returned in all its glory to Locke's Beach on Christmas morning 2022. The very first Christmas Day swim in Fenit took place on 25th December 1952 and the swim has gone from strength ever since, except for the unavoidable absence of 2020 and 2021. About 700 swimmers took the plunge in Fenit in mild weather conditions to celebrate the return of a much-loved event in the Christmas Day celebrations, as hundreds of spectators looked on from every available vantage point.

The 2022 Christmas dip really caught the imagination of the public, who were suffering from cabin fever after the two-swim absence and there was a steely determination to be in Fenit to mark seventy years of midday Christmas swims. From early morning there was a constant flow of traffic into Fenit village as people arrived early to soak up the atmosphere and to meet and greet friends. The buzz of excitement and anticipation was tangible from 11.00am onwards. Arrivals at the gathering area in the fantastic new car park were met by lively seasonal music on a mild day when the rain stayed away until the swim was done and dusted.

Members of RNLI Fenit Lifeboat Station, who hosted the swim, treated people to a variety of seasonal refreshments which were well received. The many children present enjoyed the sweets and lollipops which were on offer. Santa and Mrs Claus, in full costume, kept the expanding numbers entertained with songs and revelry before directing swimmers onto Locke's Beach at 11.45am. Everybody had lined up on the sandy beach by 11.55am and Santa and Mrs Claus led the singing of a lively rendition of Jingle Bells. Such was the exuberance of the crowd, that even Santa Claus had difficulty holding the merry swimmers in line until the midday hour. There was a vibrant countdown from ten seconds to noon. The bell was then rung for an unstoppable charge to the sea.

Even the water temperature had recovered to a comfortable eight degrees Centigrade after the artic conditions of the previous week. The swell of the crowd created a warm effervescent atmosphere on land and sea and even the 'once a year' swimmers didn't admit to feeling the cold. The majority of swimmers did the customary three charges into the sea although those who wanted to avoid the rush stayed in the water. I was in the frontline for all three charges, but I kept my head out of the water just to be on the safe side as it hadn't been too long since my combined cataract and corneal surgery on the 10th November 2022. The stewarding was magnificent and the line-up was well marshalled for all three charges. A special feature of the swim was the presence of many people home for Christmas, determined not to miss the return of Ireland's longest running swim. A large cohort of young swimmers also took the plunge.

The members of RNLI Fenit Lifeboat Station, who were on hand from early morning to make the necessary preparation for a busy day, were in position with their collection boxes from 11am and were generously supported by the large crowd. This was an opportunity for the general public to acknowledge the selfless work done by RNLI Fenit Lifeboat crew throughout the year in all weather conditions. The sizeable collection was a fitting acknowledgement of these brave volunteers.

Members of RNLI Fenit Lifeboat Station provided piping hot soup, tea, coffee and mulled wine for one and all throughout the day. The warm beverages went down a treat after the exhilarating dip. All the hard work of the organising committee came to fruition on this very special milestone. The 2022 swim in Fenit was especially memorable and, very definitely, absence made the heart grow fonder for the traditional dip. It was an honour and pleasure to have been part of it. It was just super to have the swim back after a three-year hiatus. Long may the tradition continue and may we have the health to enjoy it!

CHAPTER FORTY NINE

OUTPATIENT

My first appointment with Mr Flynn in 2023 was confirmed for Wednesday, 11th January. Once again, Mr Flynn was very pleased with everything. He said that both corneal transplants were functioning well and he put me on one drop a day in the right eye and one drop four times a day in the left eye. We spoke about the lower lid chalazion in my right eye which was flaring up at times. We discussed the option of incision and curettage and I told Mr Flynn that I was keen to proceed accordingly in the hope of eliminating the discomfort in my right eye. Subsequently, I received correspondence confirming that an appointment had been arranged for my outpatient procedure, excision of chalazion, with Mr Flynn at 10.00am on Thursday, 23rd February 2023 at the Outpatients' Department, Bon Secours Hospital, College Road, Cork.

As my appointment on the 11th January 2023 had been scheduled for 10.15am, I travelled on the 7.05am train from Tralee. When I left The Elysian after my appointment with Mr Flynn, I had time to head into the city centre for a bit of shopping during the January sales. After grabbing a bite of lunch, I walked out to Kent Station and caught the 2.25pm Dublin train. Those of us heading for Kerry changed trains at Mallow and continue our journey home. I had one more visit to make to the Bon Secours Hospital, Cork. I was hoping that would be my final visit for the foreseeable future.

On a beautiful sunny spring morning on Thursday, 23rd February 2023, my wife Sheila drove me to the Bon Secours Hospital in Cork to have the chalazion in my right eye excised. As I was due to check in at the Outpatients' Department before 10am we left home at 7.30am in case road traffic was heavy. We also allowed for any loss of time due to unexpected roadworks along our route. This was our first opportunity to travel on the recently opened Macroom bypass and both of us were very impressed with a most beautiful bit of infrastructural engineering. As well as being a pleasure to travel on it, the bypass reduced our travelling time to Cork by about twenty minutes. I'm sure the bypass has also brought great relief to the good citizens of Macroom who for many years have had to endure traffic congestion on the main street of their lovely market town. I fondly recall hitching to and from Cork during my student days in UCC. Whenever I was dropped off in Macroom, I didn't have long to wait for my next lift. Traffic was moving so slowly through the town centre that motorists were delighted with a bit of company for a chat during the snail's pace progress from one end of the town to the other. It was a great place to be picked up as the lift usually landed you in to Cork City if going one way or in to Killarney or Tralee if you were travelling in the Kerry direction. I don't know if people still hitch a lift but if they do, the new dual carriage way that bypasses Macroom won't help their cause as the traffic moves fairly lively on the fabulous new motorway.

I signed in at the Outpatients' Department at the Bon Secours Hospital at around 9.45am and was asked to take a seat in the nearby waiting room. As always, the room was full to capacity with people who were in the hospital for appointments with the consultants of different disciplines. I was called for my appointment with Mr Flynn at 10.15am. He explained how he was going to remove the goo from the eyelid. I was placed in a lying position and a local anaesthetic was administered by Mr Flynn. The entire procedure took about twenty minutes. The eye was then cleaned with an ointment and covered with a pad. I was instructed to keep the right eye dry and to keep the pad in place until 6pm. I was also given a tube of antibiotic ointment which I was to apply to the eye twice a day for one week. Mr Flynn also told me to continue applying one drop per day into the right eye and one drop three times per day into the left eye. Sheila and I then went for a late breakfast and a little shopping before driving home. My right eye was black and blue for a few days but the discomfort caused by the chalazion was now gone. After a few days normal colour had returned to my lower eyelid and the antiseptic ointment had prevented any further infection.

I had now completed four visits to Bon Secours Hospital, Cork in a ten-month period. My first corneal transplant had been performed in April 2022. I returned as an outpatient in September for the laser peripheral iridotomy on my left eye. I was back in Hospital again in November for the combined cataract surgery and corneal endothelial transplant. I returned as an outpatient in February 2023 to have the chalazion in my right eye excised. By including my cataract surgery in the right eye in December 2019, I would have had five procedures in the Bons to counteract my Fuchs Dystrophy in just over three years. Since my Fuchs Dystrophy had been diagnosed by Mr Wallace in January 2018, it had been part of my life for five years. I effectively lived with it for the first two years. Then the corrective surgeries began and they had been successful. My determination to meet the disease head on had worked to my advantage. From the beginning, I accepted that I had little choice if I didn't want to suffer a serious deterioration in my vision or even lose my sight altogether. The support of my wife, Sheila from the get go was crucial. She kept my spirits up and never allowed me to fall victim to my condition. I was very fortunate to have voluntary health insurance which allowed me to have my operations without undue delay. My full agenda as Chairman of Austin Stacks GAA Club was a welcome distraction. The success enjoyed by the Club during my term in office, especially the achievement of winning the County Senior Football Championship in 2021, drove me on to personal success with the problem in my eyes.

Above all, the return of Mr Flynn from London to Cork was my greatest blessing. It meant that I didn't have to go to Dublin or London for my surgeries. It allowed me a convenient journey by car or train for my frequent visits to the Bon Secours Hospital Cork or the Eye Clinic at the Elysian in Cork. Most importantly, I was been cared for by Mr Tom Flynn, Consultant Ophthalmic Surgeon and one of the leading specialists in cornea, cataract and laser eye surgery. For that, I will be forever grateful.

CHAPTER FIFTY

HELEN KELLER & ANNE SULLIVAN

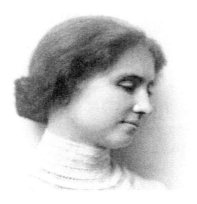

HELEN KELLER

When I was diagnosed with Fuchs Dystrophy, I was forced to face up to the fact that the good vision which I had enjoyed, indeed had taken for granted, during my life was at risk. It made me far more aware of the adjustments that people with restricted sight or no vision at all had to make in order to live a full life. I had from an early age read a great deal about Helen Keller, who lost both her sight and hearing after contracting an illness as a young child. Despite her disabilities, she lived a very full life as an author, disability rights advocate, political activist and lecturer. Helen was very fortunate when Anne Sullivan became her personal teacher from age seven. Both women became firm friends and life-long companions. Anne taught Helen how to use language, to read and to write. Helen went on to study at Perkins School for the Blind in Watertown, Massachusetts and later at Harvard University, Cambridge, Massachusetts, where she became the first deafblind person to achieve a Bachelor of Arts degree.

Helen worked for the American Foundation for the Blind for forty-five years. She travelled all over the United States as well as to thirty-five countries around the world as a determined advocate for the blind and those with restricted vision. She also published fourteen books and wrote essays and made speeches on many pressing topics of her era. Despite not being able to see or hear, she was a tireless campaigner for the disabled, for women's suffrage, for workers' rights and for world peace. She was also a founding member of the American Civil Liberties Union, a non-profit organization founded in 1920 to defend and preserve the individual rights and liberties guaranteed to every American citizen by the constitution and laws of the United States.

Helen Keller's autobiography, The Story of My Life, was published in 1903 and detailed her early life with Anne Sullivan. It was later adapted as a Broadway play and a Hollywood film. Helen dedicated her book to Alexander Graham Bell, who was one of her teachers and an advocate for the deaf. Helen's birthplace in West Tuscumbia, Alabama, USA, where she was born in 1880 was designated and preserved as a National Historic Landmark. She herself was inducted into the Alabama Women's Hall of Fame in 1971 and to the Alabama Writers' Hall of Fame in 2015.

Helen Keller suffered a number of strokes in 1961 and spent the last years of her life at her home. In 1964, President Johnson awarded her the Presidential Medal of Freedom, one of the USA's highest civilian honours. The following year she was elected to the National Women's Hall of Fame at the New York World's Fair.

Helen devoted much of her final years to raising funds for the America Foundation for the Blind. She died in her sleep on the 1st June, 1968 at her home in Easton, Connecticut, USA. After a service at the Washington National Cathedral, her remains were cremated and her ashes were buried next to her constant companion, Anne Sullivan, who was her eyes, her ears and her inspiration.

Helen Keller achieved a great deal in her long life and is an inspiration not only to disabled people but to every person who is faced with difficulties on the eventful journey through life. Being unable to see or hear she was without three of the five senses, which are sight, smell, taste, touch and hearing. Helen could have lived a lonely solitary life without seeing the beauty of the changing seasons and hearing the sound of the song birds in the sky. Instead with fortitude and resilience she accomplished more than most of us who have been blessed with the five primary senses. But even Helen Keller admitted that she could not have lived such a full life without the help of her friend and constant companion, Anne Sullivan.

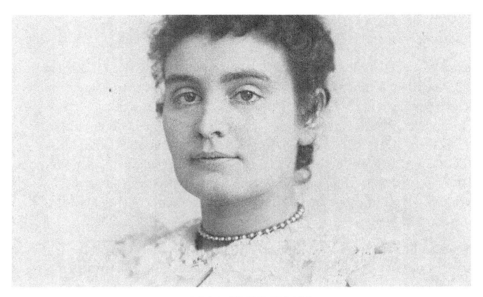

ANNE SULLIVAN

While it is widely known that Anne Sullivan was Helen Keller's teacher and companion, it is not as well known that Anne herself was partially blind. Anne was born on the 14th April 1866 in Agawam, Massachusetts, USA. At the age of five, Anne contracted the eye disease trachoma, which left her partially blind and without reading or writing skills. In 1880, Anne was admitted to Perkins School for the Blind in Watertown, Massachusetts where she learned the manual alphabet, which is a set of hand shapes that represent the letters of the alphabet. This alphabet allowed Anne to make great progress with her studies. During her time at Perkins, Anne also underwent a series of eye operations that improved her vision. Anne graduated in 1886 as the valedictorian of her class.

Shortly after Anne's graduation, the director of Perkins School for the Blind, Michael Anagnos, was contacted by Helen Keller's father, who was looking for a teacher for his seven-year-old blind and deaf daughter. Director Anagnos recommended Anne for this position and she began working as a teacher at the Kellers' home in West Tuscumbia, where she quickly connected with Helen. It was the beginning of a forty-nine-year relationship. Anne progressed from teacher to governess and finally to companion and friend.

Anne taught a vocabulary to Helen by spelling out each word out into Helen's palm. Within six months this method proved to be working well as Helen had learned 575 words, some multiplication tables and the Braille system, which is a system of raised dots that can be read with the fingers by people who are blind or who have limited vision. Anne encouraged Helen's parents to send her to the Perkins School for the Blind, where she would get an appropriate education. Once they had agreed, Anne took Helen to Boston in 1888 and stayed with her there. Anne continued to teach her bright protégée, who soon became famous for her remarkable progress. With the help of the Director Anagnos, Helen became a public symbol for the school, helping to increase its funding and donations and making it the most famous and sought-after school for the blind in the country. Anne remained a close companion to Helen and continued to assist in her education, which ultimately included her BA degree from Radcliffe College, Harvard University. Anne continued to live with Helen as her personal assistant and in 1932 they were each awarded honorary fellowships from the Education Institute of Scotland as well as honorary degrees from Temple University, Philadelphia.

Anne had been visually impaired for almost all of her life, but by 1901, after having a stroke at thirty-five years of age, she became completely blind. On the 15th October, 1936, she had a coronary thrombosis and fell into a coma. She died five days later at the age of 70 years with Helen holding her hand.

Helen Keller and Anne Sullivan were two marvellous women who achieved so much despite their separate disabilities. While Helen is the more famous of the two, Anne was a trail blazer in her own right. The two companions gave hope to blind and deafblind people throughout the world and proved that blindness and deafness can be overcome by those with determination and the support of those around them. Today, The Helen Keller Foundation for Research and Education continues the work to which Helen dedicated her life. It draws its inspiration from her achievements. Its global efforts to end blindness and deafness through medical research are as a result of Helen's belief that no matter what the obstacle anything is possible. Likewise, The Anne Sullivan Foundation for people who are Deafblind provides a range of services for people who are deafblind. It aims to support each person in their ongoing development while taking account of their individual needs and preferences.

CHAPTER FIFTY ONE

RAFTERY THE POET

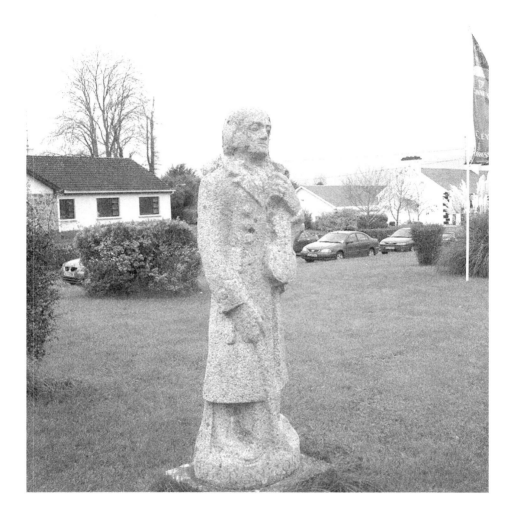

RAFTERY STATUE AT CRAUGHWELL, CO. GALWAY

Back in the day, when I was a secondary school student, I was introduced by my Irish teacher to the poetry of Anthony Raftery who conversed in his native language and was known in Irish as Antoine Ó

Raifteirí. He was the first blindman that I ever encountered, even if only in literature, and I was fascinated by his life and times. He is regarded as one of the last of the wandering bards. As a student, I assumed that Raftery was a scholarly and erudite man who had written very beautiful poetry in the Irish language. The emphasis in school was very much on learning his poetry but as I began researching his life and times, I realised that he actually had little or no formal schooling and, due to his blindness, he was more than likely illiterate.

Anthony was born in Kiltimagh, County Mayo in 1779. He was one of nine children and, by all accounts, he was an intelligent and curious child. When Anthony was about six or seven years of age, smallpox devastated his family. Within a few weeks all of his eight siblings had died and he himself was left blind.

As his father was a weaver for the local Anglo-Irish landlord Frank Taaffe, Anthony was safeguarded from the worst of the poverty of the time, but without his sight it would be much more difficult for him to earn a living as an adult. Anthony was gifted with a talent for music and poetry and went on to become one of Ireland's best known Irish language poets. He got by playing the fiddle and performing his songs and poems as he traversed the west of Ireland. He is believed to be one of the last of the travelling bards.

Like many of the poets of that era, Anthony had a patron in Frank Taaffe, who provided him with basic board and lodgings where he could write songs and poetry for the entertainment of the local gentry. Wrote is probably the wrong word to use because it's very likely that Anthony never learned to read or write because of his blindness. The bards of the time practised an oral tradition whereby they memorised their songs, poems and poetry and passed them on by word of mouth. It was many years later before Anthony's work was written down.

There is one story told, that, on a particular night, Taaffe sent Anthony and a servant to a neighbouring town to get more drink for his guests. Both men travelled on separate horses but Anthony's horse somehow left the road on the dark night, stumbled and suffered a broken neck which was fatal. Another story, which is more credible, as it is difficult to visualise a blindman riding a horse in the dark to a distant destination, suggests that Anthony wrote a particular poem to which his patron Taaffe took exception. Every bard who enjoyed patronage was expected to sing the praises of his benefactor in his work but, apparently, Anthony had been critical of the landed gentry in this particular poem.

In any event, Taaffe banished Anthony from his domain and so the itinerant life of the wandering bard commenced. He was a familiar sight on the roads in the west of Ireland, as he always wore a long frieze coat and corduroy breeches. By all accounts, he was a very strong man and a good wrestler. As well as eking out a living from his music, songs and poetry, Anthony regularly participated in the wrestling matches that were popular at the time and provided the winners with a modest purse.

But, it's for his poetry that Anthony Raftery, the blind bard is fondly remembered. None of his poems were written down during his own lifetime but they were later collected and written down by Douglas Hyde, Lady Gregory and others from those who had memorised them. Once his poems were published, they became very popular and were soon included in the formal Irish syllabus of schools.

One of Anthony's most beautiful poems is "Mise Raifteirí an File," which he frequently recited in Irish about his life as a poet. In this poem, Anthony expresses his frustration at never feeling fulfilled or rewarded fairly for his literary genius. The poem was later translated into English but it's highly likely that this was done after his death as Anthony had very little English and was totally committed to the Irish language.

Mise Raifteirí an File/I am Raftery the Poet

Mise Raifteirí an file/ I am Raftery the poet
Lán dóchas is grá/ Full of hope and love
Le súile gan solas/ With eyes without light
Le ciúnas gan chrá/ Calm without anguish

'Dul siar ar m'aistear/ Going back in my travels
Le solas mo chroí/ With the light of my heart
Fann agus tuirseach/ Weary and tired
Go deireadh mo shlí/ To the end of my journey

Féach anois mé/ Look at me now
Is mo chúl le balla/ And my back to the wall
Ag seinm ceoil/ Playing music
Do phócaí folmha/ To empty pockets

His most famous work, probably, is Anach Cuan, a lament he composed for the twenty people from Annaghdown (Anach Cuan), who drowned at Menlo, Co. Galway in 1828 while on their way to a fair in Galway. Annaghdown is a parish in County Galway which takes its name from Eanach Dhúin, the Irish for "the marsh of the fort." Apparently, about thirty villagers with sheep and other goods set out in an old boat from the Annaghdown Pier on the shores of Lough Corrib to travel the eight miles to Galway. Back in those days there was no traversable road and it was usual to travel by lake. The old boat sprung a leak a few miles from Galway. One of the men on the boat tried to plug the leak with his coat. But as he pressed it more firmly into place with his heel, his leg went through the rotten timber plank. Within second, the boat sank leaving the passengers struggling in the water. Eleven people managed to reach the safety of the nearby shore but eleven men and eight women were drowned in that awful tragedy which was immortalised by Anthony in his haunting lament. Because of the length of the lament, only the English translation follows below and the original Irish version is easily accessible online.

ANACH CUAN
If my health is spared, I'll be long relating
Of the boat that sailed out from Anach Cuan
And the keening after of mother and father
As the laying out of each corpse was done

Oh, King of Graces, who died to save us
It was a small affair but for one or two
But a boat-load bravely on a calm sailing
Without storm or rain to be swept to doom

The boat sprang a leak and left all those people

And frightened sheep out adrift on the tide
It beats all telling what fate befell them
Eleven strong men and eight women died

Men who could manage a plough or harrow
For to break the fallow or scatter seed
And the women whose fingers could move so nimbly
To spin fine linen or cloth to weave

Young boys they were lying where crops were ripening
From the strength of youth, they were borne away
In their wedding clothes for their wake they robed them
Oh, King of Glory man's hope is vain

May burning mountains come tumbling downward
On that place of drowning may curses fall
Full many the soul it has left in mourning
And left without hope of a bright day's dawn

The cause of their fate was no fault of sailing
It was the boat that failed them the Caislean Nuadh
And left me to make with a heart that's breaking
This sad lamentation for Anach Cuain

The opening lines of Anthony's poem, Cill Aodáin are among the best
know lines in Irish poetry. They are like a long sigh of relief at the end
of a long winter, conveying a feeling of exuberance at the stretch in the
evenings and a return to life and activity.

CILL AODÁIN

Anois teacht an earraigh / Now with the coming of spring
Beidh an lá ag dul chun síneadh / The days will be getting longer
'S tar éis na Féile Bríde / And after the feast of Bridget
Ardóidh mé mo sheol / I will raise my sail
Ó chuir mé i mo cheann é / Since I got it into my head
Ní chónóidh mé choíche / I will not settle

Go seasfaidh mé síos / Until I stand down
I lár Chontae Mhaigh Eo / In the middle of County Mayo

Anthony died at Killeeneen, near Craughwell, County Galway in 1835 at fifty-six years of age. He was buried in nearby Killeeneen Cemetery. In 1900, Lady Gregory, Edward Martyn and WB Yeats built a memorial stone over his grave, bearing the inscription "RAFTERY". A statue of him stands in the village green in Craughwell, opposite Cawley's pub. Like many great artists, Anthony Raftery's genius was not especially recognised in his own lifetime but posthumously he became very famous. Life at the time was very difficult for a wandering bard, but for a blind man it must have been very uncertain and dangerous as he wandered the roads. His legacy benefitted from the great oral tradition of passing down songs, stories and poetry from one generation to the next. His work will live on forever and he will always be remembered as a brilliant oral composure of poetry that gave us a look into the social history of the time and into the life of a man whose blindness didn't prevent him from living a full and productive life.

CHAPTER FIFTY TWO

THE BLIND SINGERS

As I was reading bits and pieces about Fuchs Dystrophy and blindness, I can across some very interesting material published by the Guide Dogs of Hawaii, an advocacy organisation for the blind of Hawaii. The aim of the organisation is to empower the Blind and Visually Impaired of Hawaii to conquer barriers by providing guide dog support, technology aids, mobility training, and community access to participate in everyday activities. Amongst other little gyms, the organisation's website contains a list of the ten most famous blind people in the world living or deceased. Helen Keller is listed at number eight and surprisingly the top three names on the list are singers. They are Stevie Wonder, Ray Charles and Andrea Bocelli, respectively. As I am very interested in music and song, I found that particular statistic to be confirmation of the joy and happiness which music and song brings to the lives of people of all abilities. It also proves, if proof was needed, that a handicap, however severe, can be overcome by those who have a God given talent that they wish to develop for personal career development and for sharing with wider audiences.

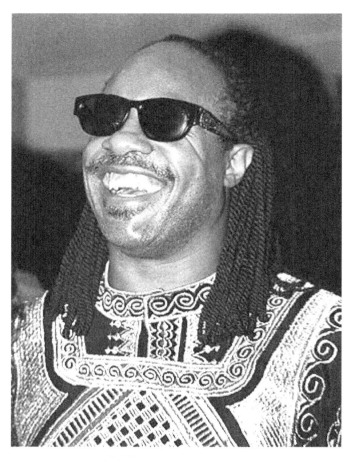

STEVIE WONDER

Stevie is an American singer-songwriter and a former child prodigy who is one of the most creative musical figures of the past sixty years with hits like *My Cherie Amour*, *You Are the Sunshine of My Life* and *Superstition*. He is credited as a pioneer and influence by musicians across a range of genres that include rhythm and blues, pop, soul, gospel, funk and jazz. He was born six weeks premature on the 13th May, 1950, in Saginaw, Michigan, USA with a condition that caused his early blindness. Despite being blind, he showed an early gift for music, first with a church choir in Detroit, Michigan and later with a range of instruments, including the harmonica, piano and drums, all of which he taught himself before he was ten years of age.

Stevie was only eleven years old when he was discovered by Ronnie White of the Motown band, The Miracles. In 1962, he released his debut *The Jazz Soul of Little Stevie Wonder*, an instrumental album that showed off his remarkable musicianship. The same year he also released *Tribute to Uncle Ray*, where Wonder covered the songs of blind soul icon Ray Charles. Stevie then developed a major following with the album *Little Stevie Wonder the 12-Year-Old Genius.*

Stevie went on to study classical piano and work on his musicianship and song writing capabilities. After dropping "Little" from his stage name in the mid-1960s, he has enjoyed decades of successful albums and singles. Among my personal favourites from the 1970's are *Shoo-Be-Doo-Be-Doo-Da-Day*, *My Cherie Amour*, *Yester-Me, Yester-You, Yesterday* and *Don't You Worry 'Bout a Thing*. In 1982, Stevie teamed up with ex-Beatle Paul McCartney for the No. 1 single *Ebony and Ivory*, a song promoting racial harmony. In 1984, he released the massive No. 1 pop single *I Just Called to Say I Love You*.

Stevie is one of the best-selling music artists of all time, with sales of over 100 million records worldwide. He has won twenty five Grammy Awards and one Academy Award for Best Original Song in the 1984 film *The Woman in Red*. He has been inducted into the Rhythm and Blues Music Hall of Fame, Rock and Roll Hall of Fame and Songwriters Hall of Fame.

Stevie is also noted for his work as an activist for political causes, including his 1980 campaign to make Martin Luther King Jr.'s birthday a federal holiday in the U.S. In 2009, he was named a United Nations Messenger of Peace, and in 2014, he was honoured with the Presidential Medal of Freedom. Steve dedicated his 1984 Oscar win to anti-apartheid activist Nelson Mandela of South Africa and also performed on the No. 1 charity singles *We Are the World*, to raise money for famine relief in Africa

Steve is a long-time advocate for improved services for the blind and those with disabilities. In connection with the International Day of Persons with Disabilities, he was named a United Nations Messenger of Peace in 2009. In June 2013, Stevie continued his advocacy work when he announced he would make good on a promise to perform a concert in Marrakech for negotiators from the World Intellectual Property Organization when they agreed on an international treaty providing blind and visually impaired individuals around the world with more access to books.

Stevie Wonder is probably the best-known blind person in the world. He is an example not only to the blind but to the disabled, in general. He never dwells on his blindness but lives his professional and private life to the full.

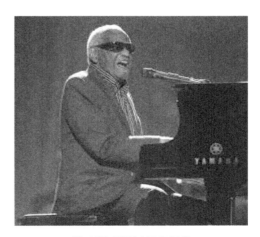

RAY CHARLES

Ray was an American singer, songwriter, pianist and alto saxophonist. He is regarded as one of the most iconic and influential singers in history, and was often referred to by his contemporaries as 'The Genius' and 'Uncle Ray.' Among friends and fellow musicians, he preferred being called 'Brother Ray.' He was born in Albany, Georgia, USA on the 23rd September 1930 and began to lose his sight at the age of five, most likely due to glaucoma. He was totally blind by the age of seven. Ray attended Florida School for the Deaf and the Blind in St. Augustine from 1937 to 1945. It was there that his musical talent was developed and he was taught to play the classical piano music of Bach, Mozart and Beethoven by his teacher, Mrs Lawrence, who also taught him how to use braille music.

After leaving school, Ray headed to Jacksonville to become a pianist in a Band. He subsequently moved on to Orlando for a while. His next move was to Los Angeles and finally to Seattle, building a reputation as a singer and pianist all along the way as well as having a few minor hit songs.

Ray pioneered the soul music genre by combining blues, jazz, rhythm and blues and gospel music and was signed by Atlantic Records. Ray's big hit in 1960, *Georgia on My Mind*, was the first of his three-career number one successes. During his time with Atlantic, Ray went on the road touring with a big band where he integrated the various genres to create major hits such as *Georgia on my Mind, Unchain My Heart* and *Hit the Road Jack*.

In 1960, Ray received his first Grammy Award for *Georgia on My Mind*, followed by another Grammy for the single *Hit the Road, Jack*. Ray broke down the boundaries of music genres in 1962 with *Modern Sounds in Country and Western Music*. On this album, he gave his own soulful interpretations of many country classics.

In 1980, Ray appeared in the comedy *The Blues Brothers* with John Belushi and Dan Aykroyd. The music icon received a special honour a few years later as one of the first people inducted into the Rock and Roll Hall of Fame. Ray returned to the spotlight in the early 1990s with several high-profile appearances. He also recorded commercials for Pepsi-Cola, singing *You Got the Right One, Baby!* as his catchphrase, and performed *We Are the World* for the organization, USA for Africa, alongside the likes of Stevie Wonder, Billy Joel, Diana Ross, Cyndi Lauper, Bruce Springsteen and Smokey Robinson.

In 2003, Ray had to cancel a tour for the first time in 53 years. He underwent hip replacement surgery. While that operation was successful, he soon learned he was suffering from liver disease. He died on the 10th June, 2004, at his home in Beverly Hills, California. During his lifetime, Ray recorded more than 60 albums and performed more than 10,000 concerts.

Despite the many difficulties in his personal life, Ray Charles was an icon for blind and disabled people. The Ray Charles Foundation was setup in 1986 to financially support institutions and organizations in the research of hearing disorders. It has provided financial donations to numerous institutions involved in hearing loss research and education. The Foundation administers funds for scientific, educational and charitable purposes. It encourages, promotes and educates about the causes and cures for diseases and disabilities of the hearing impaired.

The Foundation also assists organizations and institutions in their social educational and academic advancement of programs for the youth. The Foundation's executive offices are at the historic RPM International Building, originally the home of Ray Charles Enterprises and now also home to the Ray Charles Memorial Library on the first floor, which was founded on the 23rd September 2010. The library was founded to provide an avenue for young children to experience music and art in a way that will inspire their creativity and imagination. Its main goal is to educate mass groups of underprivileged youth and provide art and history to those without access to such documents.

Despite his blindness, Ray enjoyed playing chess. As part of his therapy when he quit heroin, he met with psychiatrist Friedrich Hacker, who taught him how to play chess. He used a special board with raised squares and holes for the pieces. When questioned if people try to cheat against a blind man, he joked in reply, "You can't cheat in chess... I'm gonna see that!" In a 1991 concert, he referred to Willie Nelson as 'my chess partner.' In 2002, he played and lost to the American grandmaster and former U.S. champion Larry Evans.

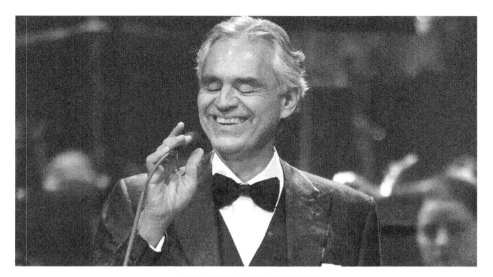

ANDREA BOCELLI

Andrea who was born on the 22nd September 1958 in Lajatico, Tuscany, Italy is an Italian tenor and multi-instrumentalist. He was born visually impaired, with congenital glaucoma and at twelve years of age, Andrea completely lost his vision due to a football accident. He was hit in the eye while playing goalkeeper during a match and experienced a brain haemorrhage. Doctors resorted to leeches in a last-ditch effort to save his sight, but they were unsuccessful and he remained blind.

Andrea spent a great deal of time singing during his childhood. He gave his first concert in a small village not far from where he was born. He won his first song competition at fourteen years of age with *O sole mio* at the Margherita d'Oro in Viareggio. He finished secondary school in 1980, and then studied law at the University of Pisa. He completed law school and spent one year as a court-appointed lawyer.

To earn money, he performed evenings in piano bars and competed in local singing competitions. He signed a recording contract with Sugar Music label and became famous in 1994 when he won the newcomer's section of the 44th San Remo Music Festival with a performance of *Il mare calmo della sera*, which was later released as his debut single.

Since 1994, Andrea has recorded fifteen solo studio albums of both pop and classical music, three greatest hits albums, and nine complete operas, selling over seventy-five million records worldwide. He has had success as a crossover performer, bringing classical music to the top of international pop charts. His album *Romanza* is one of the best-selling albums of all time, while *Sacred Arias* is the biggest selling classical album by any solo artist in history. *My Christmas* was the best-selling holiday album of 2009 and one of the best-selling holiday albums in the United States. The 2019 album *Sì* debuted at number one on the UK and USA Albums Chart, becoming Bocelli's first number-one album in both countries. His song *Con te partirò*, included on his second album *Bocelli*, is one of the best-selling singles of all time.

In 1998, Andrea was named one of People magazine's fifty most beautiful people. He duetted with Celine Dion on the song *The Prayer* for the animated film *Quest for Camelot*, which won the Golden Globe Award for Best Original Song and was nominated for the Academy Award for Best Original Song. In 1999, he was nominated for Best New Artist at the Grammy Awards. He was listed in the Guinness Book of World Records with the release of his classical album *Sacred Arias*, as he simultaneously held the top three positions on the US Classical Albums charts.

Andrea was made a Grand Officer of the Order of Merit of the Italian Republic in 2006 and was honoured with a star on the Hollywood Walk of Fame on the 2nd March 2010 for his contribution to Live Theatre. Celine Dion has said that "if God would have a singing voice, he must sound a lot like Andrea Bocelli." David Foster has often described Andrea's voice as the most beautiful in the world.

Andrea is a self-declared fan of Italian football club Inter Milan. In an interview in Pisa, he told a group of Inter Milan fans that "My passion for Inter Milan started during my college years, when Inter Milan was winning everything in Italy and the world. When Inter Milan won the Champions League in 2010, I was with my friends and I was listening to the game on the radio, and everything was a little bit in advance so I was celebrating before them. That night I was also brought to tears of joy. The treble is a feeling no one in Italy will be able to equal."

A great deal of the research at Massachusetts Institute of Technology (MIT) Boston to develop an array of new technologies to empower blind people to live, study and work more independently, is funded by the Andrea Bocelli Foundation. Andrea characterized the research as going from the "impossible to the possible by creating a tool, a device, that would basically substitute itself for the eyes."

The genesis of the Bocelli-MIT high-tech vision venture was a post-concert meeting in Boston several years ago. Andrea brainstormed with several MIT professors to find out what kind of technology for the blind would be possible. Since then, a collaborative team of cross-disciplinary researchers has developed prototypes that may someday be able to deliver critical data to the blind - everything from dynamic information about safe walking terrain and hazards, to enhancing social interactions in real-time through wearable devices or a vibrating watch with a high-resolution tactile display that can deliver important information through the skin. The Andrea Bocelli Foundation has given about €1,000,000 to fund researchers at MIT to help develop these technologies.

A central part of the MIT research is called *The Fifth Sense Project*, which is seeking to replace the missing sense of sight. It involves a team of researchers developing wearable devices for blind and low-vision people that combine sensing, computation and interaction to provide the wearer with timely, task-appropriate information about the surroundings — the kind of information that sighted people get from their visual systems, typically without conscious effort. The Fifth Sense Project focuses on three main areas:

1. Safe Mobility & Navigation
The technology tries to get at some really critical questions about safely getting around in the world, for instance, where are the appropriate walking surfaces and how can blind people avoid tripping and collision hazards? Ultimately the device might be able to answer more specific

questions, like: Where am I? Which way is it to my destination? When is the next turn, landmark or other salient environmental aspect coming up? Do my surroundings include text, and if so, what is it? Where is the kiosk, admissions desk, elevator lobby, water fountain, for instance, that I seek? What transit options such as bus, taxi, train, etc. are nearby or arriving?

2. Detecting & Identifying People
Social interactions are, obviously, essential for a full life. For the blind, it's not so easy to initiate these kinds of interactions, so the technology aims to, for example, let users know when friends, strangers or acquaintances are approaching and who they are. What is their body stance and body language? What are they wearing?

3. How to Convey Information Non-Visually Through Tactile and Aural Interfaces
The key question is how can the system effectively engage in spoken dialogue with the blind or visually impaired person so that he or she can specify goals or needs or desires? Obviously, there are already technologies out there to assist the blind.

The American Federation for the Blind identifies general items, like computers, smartphones and GPS devices, and more personally tailored devices, including everything from screen readers for blind individuals or screen magnifiers for low-vision computer users, devices for reading and writing with low vision, to braille watches and braille printers. Others have personalized devices even further, like an iPhone app that allows blind people to receive quick answers about their surroundings from sighted web volunteers who answer questions submitted over the Internet.

But the MIT team's wearable device project is more ambitious. Eventually the technology should work in real-time, they say, and support both mobility and social functions without sacrificing privacy. There is a pressing need to develop assistant technology for blind people when one realises that the unemployment rate for blind people is estimated at 75% in the United States, and almost approaches 100% in many parts of the developing world. Access to education is a key barrier as many blind and visually impaired children are simply left behind, unable to access the materials needed for their studies, especially in the areas of science, engineering and technology.

The generosity of the Andrea Bocelli Foundation in financing the Bocelli-MIT research will ensure that The Fifth Sense project will considerably improve the quality of life of the blind and the partially blind. The new technology will reduce unemployment and lead to greater inclusion of people who are deprived of the sense of sight.

When Andrea addressed an MIT workshop, to introduce new technologies to empower blind people to become more independent, he said that he was pleased to have sparked the flurry of high-tech vision research. Low-key, wearing dark sunglasses and encircled by his Italian minders, Andrea was asked if he'd be sporting a wearable device or vibrating watch someday in the future. He paused for a second, shrugged and, reverting to English replied: "Why not?" Why not indeed!

CHAPTER FIFTY THREE

VISUALLY IMPAIRED IRISH PERSONALITIES

According to The National Council for the Blind of Ireland (NCBI) there are an estimated 55,000 people in Ireland who are blind or visually impaired. There are at least 4,700 children of school-going age in Ireland who are blind or visually impaired and about 280 in higher education. The term 'visual impairment' covers moderate sight loss, severe sight loss and blindness. Age-related macular degeneration (AMD) is the leading cause of sight loss in Ireland for people over fifty years of age. There are two forms of AMD – dry AMD and wet AMD and both cause progressive sight loss.

Back in 2021, Barry Walsh writing in the Focus on Diversity website profiled a number of inspirational people with sight loss who are thriving in their careers. I have picked out a few of those visually impaired people whose disability didn't prevent them from making an impact in their fields of interest.

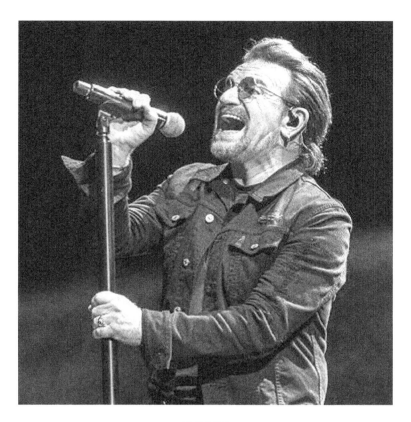

BONO

Bono – Musician
Bono has Glaucoma. He wears sunglasses indoors, which has become a trademark of his, not because he is a Diva-like individual but because of his condition. On The Graham Norton Show he stated that it was a good opportunity to explain to people that he has had glaucoma for the last twenty years. He said he has good treatments and that he is doing fine. "You're not going to get this out of your head now and you will be saying, ah, poor old visually impaired Bono," he jokingly remarked to Graham. He said his eyes are very sensitive to light. If somebody takes his photograph, he will see the flash for the rest of the day. His right eye swells up. He has a blockage so that his eyes go red a lot. He went on to add that the sunglasses are part vanity, part privacy and part sensitivity. Bono says that even though he suffers from Glaucoma it proves that

having Glaucoma doesn't mean you have to go blind. Glaucoma treatments work but, like most diseases, the earlier you get diagnosed the better, although Glaucoma may have no obvious symptoms in its early stages.

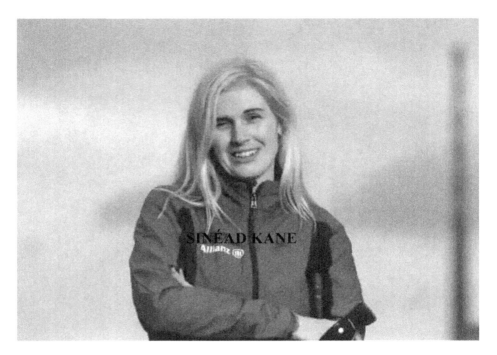

Sinéad Kane – Ultra Marathon runner
With only five percent vision since birth, Sinéad Kane is now a qualified solicitor, an ultra-Marathon runner, world record holder, keynote speaker with two Ph.Ds in law, one from Dublin City University (DCU) and the other from the National University of Ireland (NUI). Sinead along with her guide John O'Regan, completed the seven marathons on seven continents in seven days challenge, being the first visually impaired person to do so in the world. Sinead also has two world records in distance running for running 130km in 12 hours on a treadmill. She regularly speaks at conferences throughout the world.

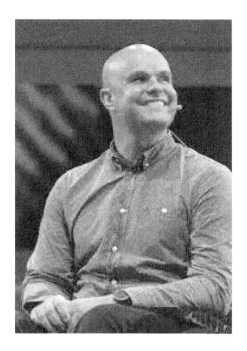

MARK POLLOCK

Mark Pollock – CEO, athlete & adventurer
Mark lost the sight in his right eye when he was five years old. Mark was about to qualify from college and take up a position in a bank in London, when, without warning he suddenly went totally blind in both eyes. Mark continued to push himself to the limit of his physical disability. He raised thousands for the charity Sightsavers by crossing the Gobi Desert, running six marathons in seven days. In 2010, Mark fell from a window of his friend's house. He broke his back and was left paralysed. Continuing his sporting challenges, Mark was awarded an honorary degree by Trinity College Dublin (TCD) and has been awarded an Honorary Doctorate from Queen's University Belfast (QUB) and The Royal College of Surgeons (RCSI). In 2012, Mark was honoured with a Rehab People of the Year Award. He has set up his own Trust and has been invited to speak at the prestigious Ted Talks, which are influential videos from expert speakers on education, business, science, tech and creativity, with subtitles in more than one hundred languages.

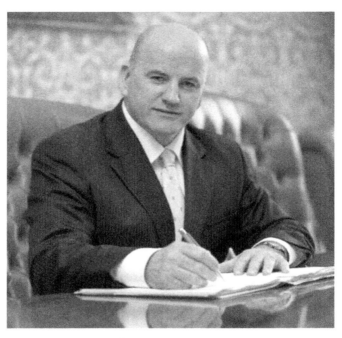

SEÁN GALLAGHER

Seán Gallagher – Investor and Politician

Sean was blind from birth as a result of congenital cataracts. He later had corrective surgery which improved his sight but he has been blind for the majority of his life. Having qualified from college, he worked with young people from the travelling community, young offenders and young people with disabilities. He was the author of the country's first National Alcohol Education Programme for the Irish Youth service. In 2002, Seán founded *Smarthomes*, a home technology business. With the success of the company, he went on to be become a self-made millionaire. In 2008, Sean featured as an investor on the RTÉ One version of Dragon's Den. He continued as an investor for three series. In 2011, he ran for the presidency of Ireland, eventually finishing second to the winner Michael D Higgins. Since then, he has worked as an advocate for those with sight loss and as a columnist in The Sunday Business Post, where he profiles an Irish start-up business each week. In August 2018, Sean again contested the election to become President of Ireland, where he finished in third place.

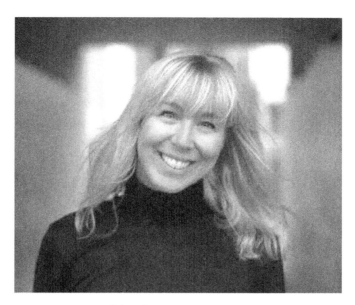

CAROLINE CASEY

Caroline Casey – CEO of The Valuable 500

Caroline was born with ocular albinism and is legally blind. At twenty-eight years of age, Caroline left her job in Accenture to launch the Aisling Foundation, which aims to improve the treatment of people with disabilities. In 2001, she trekked solo across India, raising €250k for The National Council for the Visually Impaired of Ireland and Sightsavers. She became the first western female Mahout in India. The title Mahout is bestowed in South and South East Asia on a person who works with, rides and tends an elephant. Caroline's journey across India was turned into a documentary and a TED Talk. In 2005, Caroline created O2 Ability Awards and set up the *Kanchi Foundation* in 2005 to recognise organisations that promote disability inclusion. In 2008, the foundation was renamed *Kanchi* which was the name of the elephant used on the Indian expedition. In 2017, she launched a campaign called The Valuable 500. The campaign is asking businesses to put people with disabilities on their boardroom agendas. It's also seeking to identify the next high-profile business leaders who will lead the charge for the one billion people living with disabilities worldwide.

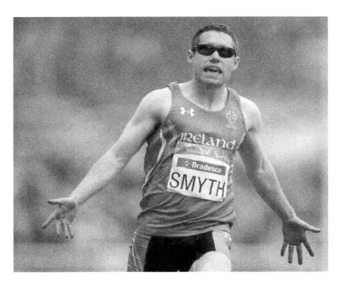

JASON SMYTH

Jason Smyth – Paralympian
Jason from Derry was born with Stargardt's Disease, which meant that he has only had ten per cent vision since birth. A Paralympian sprinter, Jason has competed in three paralympic games, winning six gold medals. He also competed for Northern Ireland in the fully-abled Commonwealth Games. Jason holds the world record in all of the Paralympics events he has competed in. In total, Jason has won seventeen para-sports gold medals in sprinting and is known as the Usain Bolt of para-sprinting. Jason is also a motivational speaker who believes that there are no limits to what can be achieved. He maintains that success comes to those who are willing to push themselves to places where others are unwilling to go. Jason says that we all have talents but that our potential is reached only when we work hard to fulfil it. On the track it has been his mission to push the boundaries of what is possible by bridging the gap between Para sport and mainstream sport. He also works hard off the track in assisting people of all abilities to bridge their own gaps. Jason is also a brand ambassador for Sport Ireland, Northern Ireland Sport and Allianz Insurance. In March 2023, Jason announced his retirement from competitive sport at the age of thirty-five, having remained unbeaten in a para-athletics career which

began at the 2005 European Games. Jason will continue to be a hugely positive influence on Irish Paralympic Sport away from the track as he has joined the staff at Paralympics Ireland as Strategy Manager with the organisation.

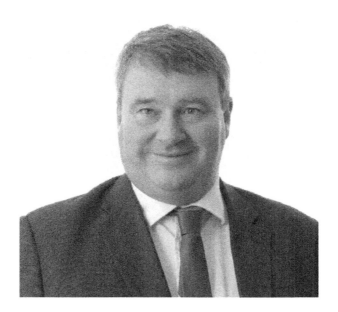

SENATOR MARTIN CONWAY

Senator Martin Conway – Politician and Founder
Born blind, Martin had a pioneering operation on his eye-sight when he was six months old. He was born with congenital cataracts, as was his father and his grandfather. Martin realised he was 'different' when he was travelling up to Dublin by rail for a medical check-up. He told his dad that he would like to be a train driver when he grew up, but his dad pointed out that a job as a train driver wouldn't be possible because Martin's eyesight was so poor. Up to 2011, Martin had twelve operations on his eye-sight and now has 20% vision. Having studied for a BA in Politics and Economics at University College Dublin (UCD), Martin joined the family business in Ennistymon, Co Clare. Martin is a founding member of AHEAD, an independent non-profit organisation working to create inclusive environments in education and employment

for people with disabilities. The main focus of its work is further education and training, higher education and graduate employment. He is particularly proud of the Willing Able Mentoring (WAM) programme which has successfully placed over 250 graduates with disabilities in employment. In 2004, Martin was elected to Clare County Council. In 2011, he was elected to the Seanad Eireann becoming the first visually impaired person in Ireland to be elected to The Houses of the Oireachtas. Martin was then appointed the Fine Gael spokesman in the Senate on Equality and Disability.

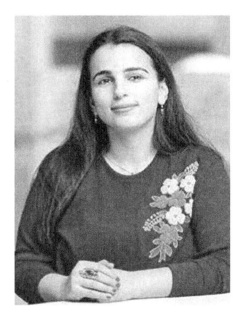

ELIONA GJECAJ

Eliona Gjecaj – statutory advisory committee of UNCRPD
Born in Albania, Eliona moved to Ireland as a child with her family. She went on to obtain a First-Class Honours Degree in International and Comparative Disability Law and Policy and a First-Class Honours BA International Studies Degree, from the University of Galway. Eliona has been recognised as 1 out of 10 Outstanding Young People of Ireland 2018 by Junior Chambers Ireland (JCI), for her disability activism, achievements, and volunteering with disability Non-Governmental

Organisations (NGO). Eliona has been Chairperson of Galway Visually Impaired Activity Club since 2016. In 2017 she was a founding member of and currently audits the Impact Society, which provides young people, and those that support them, with the social and emotional tools that are proven to help youth of any background and risk level, to develop the positive mental health required to properly navigate risk. After starting the society, Eliona ensured that a new position of Disability Officer in the Students Union of the University of Galway was established. Eliona has since gone on to be involved with the Students Union of Ireland demanding issues such as mental health, advocacy and activism be addressed within the Irish education system. Eliona was recently one of eleven people to serve on the first ever statutory advisory committee in Ireland to support monitoring of Ireland's implementation of the UN Convention on the Rights of Persons with Disabilities (UNCRPD).

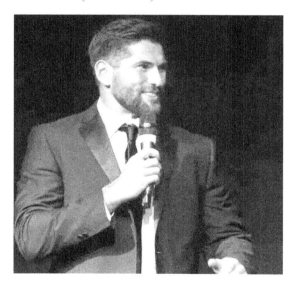

IAN MCKINLEY

Ian McKinley – Rugby Player
Ian was playing for UCD Rugby Football Club (RFC) in 2010 when a stud from a boot accidentally caught and damaged his left eye. He regained 70% vision in the eye and returned to win six caps for the

Leinster rugby team. Later that year, when he stopped at a traffic light, he said that one moment he could see the traffic light through his left eye, then in the next moment his vision went completely. Unfortunately, his retina had detached eighteen months after the initial accident and that ended his playing career at twenty-one years of age. He then moved to Italy to coach and began to play rugby again. He visited Johnny Merrigan, a researcher and lecturer at the Irish National College of Art and Design (NCAD). Johnny developed a set of protective rugby goggles to get Ian back playing. Having adjusted his game, Ian returned to the pitch, playing with his modified glasses in 2014. In 2017, Ian was called into the Italian Rugby squad qualifying under residency rules. Ian made his debut for Italy against Fiji in 2017 and won eight caps for his adopted country. Ian is now the backs coach at Rainey RCF and has not officially retired from playing. His ambition is to move into coaching as a career.

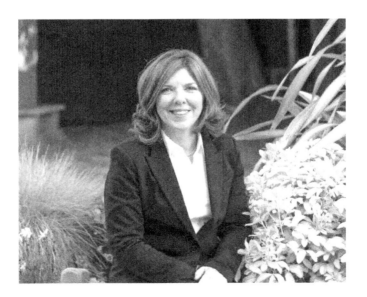

CLAIRE KENNELLY

Claire Kennelly – CEO
Claire is the founder and CEO of Inclusive World training (IWT). She is vision impaired and is personally and professionally passionate about

disability employment inclusion. Claire graduated from University College Cork (UCC) with a Bachelor of Arts (BA) degree and a Higher Diploma in Education (HDE). Claire worked for more than thirty years in all levels of the Irish education sector, including post primary, further education and higher education. In these various roles, she worked with students with varying disabilities, neuro-diversities and mental health issues. She noticed that while the students were doing well in education, they met obstacles when looking for work placement and employment. Although there are supports in place for students with disabilities to find work, there is an issue when these students try to get employment, due to the lack of inclusivity, particularly in the private sector.

Claire then set up IWT to bridge the disability employment gap between the education and private sector by showing the private sector the inclusive tools they can implement to make their workforce more diverse. IWT aims to develop disability confidence in business, community and society and thus empower young disabled people to navigate and overcome the obstacles to employment.

Claire is also the founder and presenter of the Disrupt-Ability podcast which is an education and information platform for stakeholders, including employers, employees, professionals, parents and guardians. Interviews with disabled people, advocates and activists highlight the barriers and opportunities for employing people with disabilities in Irish society and beyond. Clare's professional goal is to make Ireland a leader in employment inclusion on the global stage.

I have been very impressed by the leadership roles that people who are blind or visually impaired are taking in all walks of society. Many of them have also established or are involved with a whole variety of associations which provide support structures for blind and visually impaired people. It leads me to believe that the same can be said about other sensory disabilities such as hearing and speech disabilities.

Many people who have sensory or other disabilities are living full lives in a private capacity. It's reassuring to learn that they aren't ploughing a lone furrow. On the contrary, there are many philanthropists as well as Government and Non-Government-Organisation's (NGO) that have the best interests of the disabled at heart. During my battle with Fuchs Dystrophy, I read a great deal about blindness and visual impairment and my awareness of disability, in general, was considerably heightened. I hope that by recording my journey to save my eyesight, I have helped to ensure that the Blind and Visually Impaired will always have the supports and facilities available to enable them to live full and productive lives.

CHAPTER FIFTY FOUR

NATIONAL COUNCIL FOR THE BLIND OF IRELAND

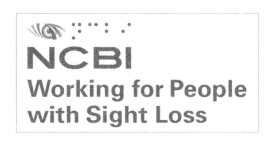

The National Council for the Welfare of the Blind of Ireland was founded on the 10th March 1931, in the Standard Hotel, Harcourt Street, Dublin. Not only was it the first voluntary body dealing with a disability group in the Irish Free State, but it set precedents in the provision of welfare and educational advancement for disadvantaged people in Ireland. The principal founders included Alice Stanley Armitage among others. The early services included home visits to poor older blind persons, home teaching service, Braille and handicrafts and referral to other charities for financial aid.

In 1935, the name was changed to the National Council for the Blind of Ireland (NCBI), which has operated nationwide since its conception in multiple settings. This ranged from NCBI sharing premises with other charities like the St. Vincent de Paul Society or operating from the teachers' homes or the homes of the Branch Chairperson or Secretary, from the parish or church-related venues, or later from the Health Board venues. In 1987, NCBI moved its Head Office to what was known as the Drumcondra Hospital on Whitworth Road, Drumcondra, Dublin 9. Since then, this permanent base together with its regional offices across the country ensures that anyone who is blind or vision impaired can have access to quality services, programmes and supports.

The National Council for the Blind of Ireland, is now the country's leading sight loss charity serving approximately 55,000 people, who are blind or vision impaired, to live confidently and independently. Its range of programmes provides practical and emotional support, rehabilitation and opening pathways to education, employment, and full participation in community and public life. It continues to raise public awareness to ensure children and adults with a significant sight loss have the same opportunities, rights, and choices as anyone else in society. NCBI works every day across the country with people of all ages, from young babies through to older members of the community. NCBI provides services to approximately 7,000 people each year.

Often when a person learns that they or a loved one, such as a parent, child or partner, is losing their sight, they have a lot of questions and fears. They are faced with a new version of their life, which initially seems limited and scary. NCBI empowers those living with sight loss in several meaningful ways to enable them to continue living independent and fulfilling lives. NCBI plays a crucial role in creating a world without barriers for people with sight loss and it endeavours to support, educate and change how people see sight loss in Ireland.

As part of its 90th year celebrations, NCBI launched a new strategic plan *Your Ambition, Our Mission 2021-2023*. The plan has partnership, innovation and service excellence at its core as it aims to improve equality of access for people who are blind or vision impaired in all aspects of their lives. It guides the organisation to be a stronger advocate for and be more relevant to and responsive to the lives of people living with sight loss.

Its vision is for people who are blind and vision-impaired to have the same opportunities, rights and choices as others to fully participate in society. Its mission is to enable people who are blind and vision impaired to overcome the barriers that impede their independence and participation in society. NCBI's core values give effect to its vision and permeates its mission and informs all of its actions to ensure that it achieves the highest standards in everything it does.

NCBI listens to people who use its services, staff members, volunteers and all other stakeholders. It collaborates with them in the design and delivery of its services and all related activities. NCBI acknowledges and respects the right of people to make choices about their lives. NCBI does everything in its power to support people who are blind and vision impaired in exercising this right.

NCBI carries out its work in an open manner and is accountable to all stakeholders for its actions and decisions. NCBI is committed to attaining excellence in everything it does through its policies, procedures and staff.

Inspired by the determination to overcome any obstacle, NCBI transforms the lives of people who are blind or vision impaired to deliver tangible change to today's needs. It offers timely information and support, relevant technology and innovative programmes to sustain those with a vision impairment in education, in the workplace, and in wider society.

Whether people are young or old, blind or vision impaired, NCBI is available to support, empower, train and advise them on all aspects of their sight loss. From birth right through to higher education, NCBI *Children and Young Person's Services* supports the development and independence of all children who are blind or vision impaired. NCBI *Adult Services* provide a diverse range of programmes and services which are designed to enable, empower and support adults to live their lives confidently and independently. NCBI's *Everyday Living Services* support people to stay connected to their local communities, to participate in leisure activities, to understand their entitlements and to maintain their enjoyment of reading. NCBI's Technology Services are designed to advise, upskill and train people on making technology (equipment, Apps, software etc.) as accessible as possible for them.

The 2016 Census of Population shows that there are 54,810 people in Ireland who are blind or vision impaired and the number is rising as the population ages. When that figure is first presented to people, usually the automatic assumption is that the majority of those people are blind, but that is not the case. Of the 55,000 or so people in Ireland who are blind or vision impaired, just 5% or approximately 2,750 of those are blind.

This means that approximately 52,250 people across the country have a form of vision impairment or are affected by sight loss in some way. The impact of vision impairment varies from person to person. Some people may be able to continue their lives as normal with their residual vision, while other people will require training, support, and more, to adapt to losing significant aspects of their vision.

One aspect of vision impairment that is often misunderstood, or not understood at all, by people who haven't experienced sight loss, is that not all vision impairment affects a person's sight in the same way. There are many different types of eye conditions that lead to vision impairment and each of those conditions affects a person's field of vision in different ways. Residual vision can be further impacted by outside influences, including lighting.

Age-related macular degeneration (AMD) is the leading cause of sight loss in Ireland for people over the age of 50. There are two forms of AMD, dry AMD and wet AMD, both of which cause progressive sight loss. There are a number of symptoms of AMD that affect vision, including distortion, where straight lines appear wavy. As the condition progresses, it can lead to the loss of a person's central vision, leaving only peripheral vision available. The symptoms and type of sight loss for a person with AMD are completely different to the symptoms and type of sight loss experienced by a person who has Glaucoma, for example.

I myself was diagnosed with one of the most serious forms of eye disease called Fuchs Dystrophy, which leads to blindness unless one undergoes corneal transplantation. In my case it meant surgeries to remove the cataracts from both my eyes and a corneal transplant of donor organ in each of my eyes. As I mentioned early, I was fortunate enough to have health insurance which allowed me to have treatment privately. I shudder to think of what may have happened if I had to await treatment in the public health service.

A large number of people are currently waiting for outpatient ophthalmic services. Figures from August 2022 from the National Treatment Purchase Fund (NTPF) data recorded that 46,310 adults were people were on waiting lists for ophthalmic services. 37,449 of those were waiting on outpatient appointments and 8,861 of those were waiting on inpatient or day case appointments. There were also 6,126 children on waiting lists for ophthalmic service. 5,508 were waiting on outpatient appointments and 618 were inpatient or day case appointments. This means that in August 2022, there was a total of 52,436 people on waiting lists for ophthalmic services.

In a bid to cut down the number of people on waiting lists and the wait time for appointments, NCBI has been continually campaigning for increased recruitment across the ophthalmology sector in Ireland. There is a shortage in the number of consultants in this field in Ireland, which is leading to waiting list issues. With such long delays for appointments, diagnosis and treatment, adults and children who are experiencing sight loss run the risk of longer-term and potentially irreversible damage to their sight.

Maintaining and maximising a person's independence is central to all NCBI's services and ensuring their active participation, retention or return to the labour market is a crucial part of this. Being in employment or self-employment boosts financial independence, mental health and social interactions. The Census shows the level of labour force participation amongst people who are blind or vision impaired in Ireland is only 24.5%. This figure means less than one person out of every four people with impaired vision are currently actively participating in the labour force. People with vision impairment have a 60% less chance of being in employment than the general population.

NCBI has a dedicated service for children and young people with vision loss that works to reduce the impact of vision loss on early development, learning and independence skills. Census 2016 figures show that since 2011, there has been a 20% increase in the number of children with vision impairment, which equates to 4,701 children of school-going age. An increasing number of children and their families are supported by NCBI each year, including 1,225 supported in 2021. This trend highlights the need for a more structured and equipped educational system, which is well positioned to support children and young adults to fulfil their potential across our educational systems.

Evidence from AHEAD, the organisation aiming to create inclusive environments in education and employment for people with disabilities, shows the extremely low representation of students who are blind or vision impaired in higher education. The participation rate has been reducing over the past number of years from 1.8% in 2015/2016 to 1.6% in 2019/2022. On paper, Disability Access Route to Education (DARE) should be improving access to third level education for young people with a vision impairment but in practice, it is not achieving that goal. NCBI recently released its Equitable Education report which focuses on strategic developments required to support children and young people who are blind or vision impaired to become independent active agents in their futures.

NCBI stresses that it's important that we have all the facts when we talk about sight loss, but it is also important that we work to dispel any age-old myths about sight loss that may be damaging or disrespectful to people who are blind or vision impaired. NCBI recently launched an online campaign called *Debunking Sight Loss Myths*, where it challenged perceptions that some people may have about sight loss. This campaign consisted of six dedicated blog posts and six dedicated posts and advertising across NCBI's social media channels. The campaign was targeted toward people who may not ordinarily be engaged with or who may not know about the work that NCBI does with the sight loss community.

NCBI's Head Office and regional centres around the country are open from 9am to 5pm from Monday to Friday each week. All relevant information about the work of NCBI can be found on its excellent website, www.ncbi.ie.

CHAPTER FIFTY FIVE

IRISH GUIDE DOGS FOR THE BLIND

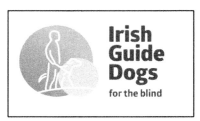

Irish Guide Dogs for the Blind is Ireland's national charity dedicated to enabling people who are visually impaired and families of children with autism to achieve improved mobility and independence. For over forty years, Irish Guide Dogs for the Blind has worked with its community of Breeders, Puppy Raisers, Home Socialisers, Temporary Boarders, Trainers, Staff, Volunteers and supporters to change as many lives as possible. Irish Guide Dogs for the Blind currently has nearly four hundred Guide and Assistance Dogs Clients in Ireland. All of its services are provided free of charge. It costs over €5 million to run the organisation each year. Over 85% of Irish Guide Dogs for the Blind's income is generated by voluntary donations and fundraising through its Branch network across the country. Soccer star, Roy Keane who is Irish Guide Dogs for the Blind's Brand Ambassador said that, having spoken to so many Guide and Assistance Dog Owners over the years, he is amazed to see what the dogs do and by the impact they have on individuals and their families. Roy added that the Guide and Assistance dogs are giving people back their lives.

Irish Guide Dogs for the Blind, which was established in 1976, has its headquarters and national training centre at Carrigrohane, Model Farm Road, Cork. It is a registered and trusted charity which provides life-changing services and supports to people who are visually impaired and to families of children with autism. It fully complies with the legislation governing Irish charities and with the relevant regulatory frameworks.

In less than two years, Irish Guide Dogs for the Blind's amazing puppies become some of the most responsible dogs in the country. Irish Guide Dogs for the Blind provides a guide through the life of a Guide Dog or Assistance Dog from puppy to retirement. Irish Guide Dogs for the Blind puppies begin life with their mother, called a Brood Bitch, in the home of one of its volunteer breeding families. By breeding its own dogs, Irish Guide Dogs for the Blind can ensure that the dogs have the best temperament and characteristics. Each puppy is introduced to various environmental stimuli in a controlled and secure way to allow the puppy to develop coping skills and to encourage the pup's confidence to grow. All of Irish Guide Dogs for the Blind's litters are organised alphabetically. The puppies in each litter are then given a name that starts with the litter's letter.

At the end of seven or eight weeks the puppies leave the homes of the volunteer breeding families. They are placed in pairs in volunteer homes for approximately a week to continue their early socialisation programme which supports their development. The pups learn to overcome obstacles like stairs, sleeping away from mum and siblings and travelling in a car. At the end of this period, puppies return to Irish Guide Dogs for the Blind's National Training Centre for puppy evaluation and are placed into puppy raisers' homes the same day.

Puppies move in with their puppy raiser family for approximately ten months, learning critical skills that will help them in their future training as Guide or Assistance Dogs such as socialisation, obedience and toilet training. The puppy learns to be confident and happy in a variety of settings e.g., busy town conditions and on quiet country roads, taking it into shops and railway stations, travelling on buses and trains and getting into lifts. The puppy also needs to be able to cope with heavy traffic, road works, and loud noises, to behave well in restaurants, church, and generally learning to deal with every situation.

Between thirteen to nineteen months and now fully grown, the puppies leave their puppy raiser family and return to Irish Guide Dogs for the Blind's National Training Centre for their technical training. They start off learning things like clicker training and how to cross roads, to stop at kerbs and how to avoid obstacles that would cause problems for its owner. If the dog reaches the high standards needed to be a Guide or Assistance Dog, it will progress to another three months of advanced training. Here the instructor perfects the dog's skills so that it can provide safe mobility for a visually impaired person. The instructor will look at how the dog behaves, its personality, whether it walks fast or slow, whether it prefers working in the country or city. From these traits the dog is matched with somebody on Irish Guide Dogs for the Blind's waiting list, who suits this particular type of dog. Getting the dog/owner match right is crucial and a lot of time and effort is put in to ensure that the best possible partnership is made.

From nineteen months onwards, once a match is made, the client attends a residential training course at Irish Guide Dog for the Blind's National Training Centre with their dog. The person returns home with their Guide Dog or Assistance Dog with new found mobility, independence and freedom. Once the dog and their owner go back to their own home, one of the Irish Guide Dogs for the Blind's instructors will visit to make sure they are both working well together and will help them to get to know different routes that the owner would make regularly, such as to work or shopping.

A working dog is normally retired after about ten years. This is a very difficult time for both dog and owner as they will have spent many years together. Sometimes the Guide or Assistance Dog owner will keep their dog as a pet for the remainder of its life. If they can't, Irish Guide Dogs for the Blind will always find a suitable home for these amazing dogs. The welfare of the dog is Irish Guide Dogs for the Blind's first priority when rehoming a dog. The owner is then trained with a new Guide or Assistance Dog as soon as possible.

People who are in a position to do so, are requested to consider donating to support the work of Irish Guide Dogs for the Blind. No matter how big or small, ever donation helps change lives. There are various ways to make a donation to Irish Guide Dogs for the Blind. For each donation of €250 or more in a given year, Irish Guide Dogs for the Blind can claim an extra 45% of that donation in tax relief at no extra cost to the donor. This simple step takes just a moment of the donor's time and nothing more. Unlocking this extra funding is vital to the people who rely on the services of Irish Guide Dogs for the Blind and for the many more it hopes to assist in the coming years.

Many families like to celebrate their loved one's life by asking friends, neighbours and colleagues to make a charitable donation instead of sending flowers. *A Gift in Memory* is a perfect tribute as well as hopefully giving great comfort in knowing that the generous gift is helping to change someone's life. All gifts, no matter how small, are greatly valued and significantly help Irish Guide Dogs for the Blind to deliver its services free of charge to those who really need them. A person can choose to make a lasting gift by having an in-memory collection at the funeral service, which can be organised by the funeral directors. In the death notice a request can be made to people to donate an in-memory gift to Irish Guide Dogs for the Blind. A person can also set up a regular in-memory gift to mark an anniversary or birthday of a loved one.

It may not be widely known that the training of one in every three Guide or Assistance Dogs is funded by legacies. A gift in a person's will can transform the lives of blind or visually impaired people and the families of children with autism. Leaving a life-changing gift in a will is an amazing act of kindness and will be most appreciated by all who will be helped as a result. A person's gift is greatly valued and helps the Irish Guide Dogs for the Blind to continue its vital work.

Many of the great strides Irish Guide Dogs for the Blind has made are thanks to the gifts left to it by people in their wills. To find out more about how these gifts change lives give Irish Guide Dogs for the Blind a call. People are also very welcome to visit Irish Council for the Blind at its National Headquarters and Training Centre in Cork to get a better understanding of its work and impacts. Once a person decides to leave a gift in a will, it is simple to implement. With a little help from a solicitor, a person simply puts a clause in the will in favour of Irish Guide Dogs for the Blind. That will ensure that the gift will reach Irish Guide Dogs for the Blind at a future date. The donation will help blind and visually impaired people achieve independence and a better quality of life.

A person can sponsor a puppy in training for as little as €10 a month. It's a great feeling to watch a puppy grow from a six-week-old bundle of fur to a fully-qualified Guide or Assistance Dog. It's a great way to support the work of Irish Guide Dogs for the Blind. After twenty-four months of training, the sponsored puppy will give freedom and independence to someone with sight loss. Each person who sponsors a puppy will receive a *pupdate* via mail or email, a personalised certificate, an adorable car sticker and pen.

Irish Guide Dogs for the Blind relies on donations to continue its life-changing work. Every euro raised makes a difference to people in Ireland living with a visual impairment and the families of children with autism. There are approximately 55,000 people in Ireland who are blind or visually impaired and the number is rising as the population ages.

As well as its Headquarters and National Training Centre in Cork, Irish Guide Dogs for the Blind has branches throughout Ireland. There is a font of very interesting information on its excellent website, www.guidedoge.ie and Irish Guide Dogs for the Blind can be contacted directly by email at info@guidedogs.ie.

CHAPTER FIFTY SIX

INEQUALITY, DISABILITY & KINDNESS

As I mentioned earlier, I have been blessed in life with good health. I have never spent much time in hospital other than for tonsilitis, appendicitis and a leg injury which I suffered during my student days in Cork. During my entire working life, I rarely missed a day off work because of illness. As well as that, I have lived a healthy lifestyle by participating in competitive sport and, when I grew a little bit older, by taking regular aerobic exercise. I have a life-long passion for sea swimming, which gives me a huge mental and physical lift. It's a form of exercise that I would highly recommend as it allows each person to swim or bathe within one's personal comfort zone. I was very competitive when I participated in swimming competitions but I would now describe myself as an aerobic swimmer, who goes with the flow, if you'll excuse the pun. I never know from day to day how long I will remain in the water until I actually get into the sea. Some days, I'm as comfortable as a fish in water while on other days every stroke is a major physical effort if my body doesn't relax as I tread water. But whether I am in the sea for a long or a short period, I never fail to feel a sense of wellbeing and serenity.

I also enjoy doing a bit of cooking. I'll be first to admit that I haven't an adventurous palate and I have a strong preference for Irish ingredients. Despite the endless attempts by my family and friend to convert me to other cuisines, I'm not for turning. I know what I like and I know what's good for me. I'm a firm supporter of home country vegetables, potatoes, fish and some meat dishes. My one occasional concession to myself is a desert of ice cream and apple pie. Overall, I maintain a simple but healthy diet and I don't take food as seriously as some of the master chefs, who make a meal out of putting a dinner on the table.

I have always believed that life is for living and there is a big difference between staying alive and living the life you have to the full. As I look back, I have few regrets. I didn't succeed in everything I did, but I always gave it my best shot and never worried about not succeeding. I have no fear of failure. Even the supreme Kerry football genius, David Clifford has been known to miss the occasional free kick although his next effort invariably ends up in the back of the net. My good friend, the late Séamus McConville, who was Editor of The Kerryman Newspaper and who first introduced me to the joy of writing, regularly described me as 'positive, persistent and tenacious' in character. Séamus read me like a good book and I certainly needed those qualities when I was diagnosed with Fuchs Dystrophy.

My battle with Fuchs Dystrophy opened my eyes – sorry! - to serious illness and disability. I have always made nominal donations to a few charitable organisations such as Disabled Artists Association, Cork, St John of God Hospitaller Services Group, The Anne Sullivan Foundation for People who are Deafblind and the Father Aurelius Maschio Salesian Missionary in India, not for any noble or philanthropic reason but because they approached me for a contribution when I began working. I was also an active member of the Saint Vincent De Paul Society for some years where I made weekly visits to people in need. Many of the people I visited were short of income or food or some of the other bare necessities of life. Some were elderly, some were unwell, some had a disability. It was a rare privilege to visit these people in their homes, to sit down for a cup of tea with them or simply spent a few minutes in chat. Their dignity in a time of need and their gratitude for the small weekly contribution given to them by the SVP made me feel inadequate at times. Sometimes, I wondered how our wealthy country could allow these fine people to go without.

When I was staring blindness straight in the face, I saw real inequality. I came to realise that those who are dependent on the public health system can be waiting for years to see a specialist. A young child with an eye problem might have a two year wait for an optical diagnosis. Everybody knows the story of people going to Belfast for cataract surgery. They, in some way, are fortunate that they have the cash in hand to pay on the day for the surgery. They can reclaim their costs from the Government but what about those who don't have the money to go to places like Belfast. Even, with a medical card, the delay is considerable. God only knows who long a patient has to wait for a corneal transplant of donor organ in the public health system.

It was clearly pointed out to me when I began my battle with Fuchs Dystrophy in an effort to save my vision, that availing of my voluntary health entitlements would not be a case of jumping the queue. It's as if the public and private health care systems are totally independent of each other. The reality is that they are. Those with health insurance and those who have the financial wherewithal to pay can avail of private health care without undue delay. Those who can't, have no option other than to join a lengthy queue. It's the way the Irish health system works but that's poor consolation to a mother whose child is in urgent need of a psychological test or medical procedure. I don't know what can be done to provide universal health care in Ireland but the dual system does cause me some concern.

Not having to worry about the cost of my own surgical procedures allowed me to approach them with the positivity, persistence and tenacity that Séamus McConville attributed to me. I was able to apply myself, without distraction, to meeting the Fuchs Dystrophy head on, to approaching each surgery with a total focus on a positive outcome and to following the post-operative guidelines that would take me further along the road to sight retention.

All I can do is wish the same for every other person in need of medical intervention. It's probably wishful thinking as inequality is as old as the world itself. Nowadays, advanced communication systems have made us more aware of inequality issues in all sectors of modern society. Solving inequality is on the agenda and there is a willingness to address it. That is a major step in the right direction.

My battle with Fuchs Dystrophy also increased my awareness of disability. During my working life as a Career Guidance Counsellor, I regular encountered students who had an educational disability and made interventions on their behalf. Psychometric diagnostic tests are available to identify various educational disabilities such as dyslexia and dyspraxia, which entitle the young people concerned to certain exemptions and concessions in the State examinations. The Central Application Office (CAO) provides the Disability Access Route to Education (DARE) which includes a range of supports for third level college applicants who have a certified educational or medical condition. Having spent a working lifetime in education, I have never been less than impressed by the Department of Education's commitment to levelling the playing field for young people with disabilities. The range of supports available to people at all levels of education ensures that people with disabilities can aspire to achieving prestigious qualifications and go on to participate fully in the world of work.

As I researched Fuchs Dystrophy and issues around illness of the eyes, I was flabbergasted by the contributions that so many blind and visually impaired people are making to society in general. I have already highlighted a few of those who have become well-known and famous because of their successful careers and special talents. They are an inspiration to all of us, not only those of us with a visual impairment but every person throughout the world who is categorised as disabled.

I am now far more aware of organisations, such as the NCBI and Irish Guide Dogs for the Blind, that advocate so effectively for the blind and visually impaired. I am more conscious of the supports that are in place to help disabled people to live full lives. Simple things like not parking in a restricted parking spot, not obstructing a footpath, providing an access ramp or a disability friendly swimming pool make a huge difference to the enjoyment of life and social inclusion of disabled people. I am also very impressed by the care, consideration and kindness shown by members of the public to disabled people.

I have first-hand experience of the dedication, empathy, care and patient centred approach of our medical professionals. Every patient is a special individual whose treatment and care are central to the work of the medical team. Having been in Hospital on a number of occasions during the recent past and having attended regularly at appointments with my medical specialists, I can say with total conviction that my battle with Fuchs Dystrophy was considerably aided by the support and kindness I received along every step of the journey. From my very first appointment with Mr Flynn when I was uncertain, apprehensive and scared of what lay ahead, I grew more confident about a successful outcome. During the years that followed, Mr Flynn and the team at the Eye Clinic in the Elysian, Cork, the staff at the Bon Secours Hospital, Cork and, of course, Dr Tom O'Regan and the team at Fairies Cross Medical Centre, Clounalour, Tralee were never less than kindness itself.

From Fenit bathing slip to the High Court
A five year journey of honour!

Billy Ryle

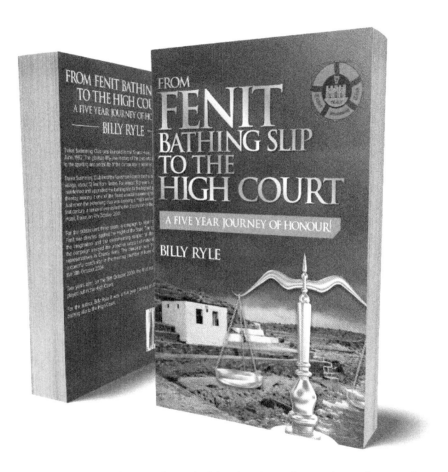

Tralee Swimming Club was founded in the Grand Hotel, Tralee on the 21st June, 1952. The glorious fifty-year history of the club and its pivotal position in the sporting and social life of the community is outlined in this book.

Tralee Swimming Club held the foreshore licence for the bathing slip at Fenit village, about 12 km from Tralee. For almost fifty years, the swimming club maintained and upgraded the bathing slip to the highest possible standard, thereby making it one of the finest coastal swimming facilities in Europe. Just when the swimming club was enjoying a major revival at the end of the last century, a series of events led to the dissolution of the club at the Grand Hotel, Tralee, on 4th October 2001.

For the subsequent three years, a campaign to retain the bathing slip in Fenit was directed against the might of the State. The campaign captured the imagination and the overwhelming support of the public. Crucially, the campaign enjoyed the proactive support of national and local public representatives in County Kerry. The campaign was finally brought to a successful conclusion in the meeting chamber of Kerry County Council on the 18th October 2004.

Two years later, on the 16th October 2006, the final act in the drama was played out in the High Court. For the author, Billy Ryle it was a five years journey of honour from Fenit bathing slip to the High Court.

AVAILABLE FOR PURCHASE ONLINE FROM BILLY RYLE
at rylebilly@gmail.com

PRICE: €15, including package & postage

Christian Brotherly Love

Billy Ryle

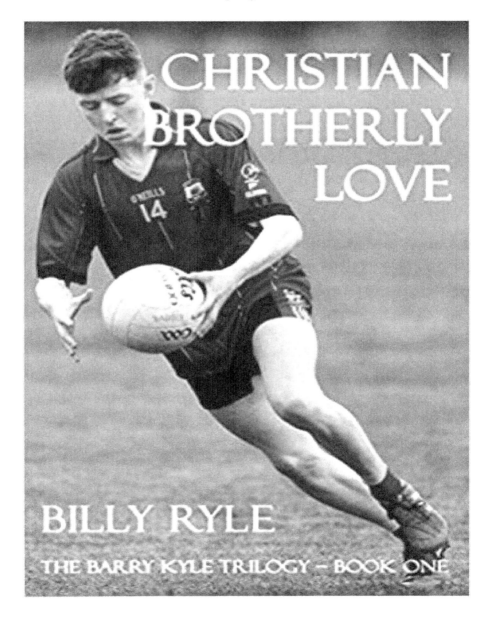

Barry Kyle, talented footballer, keen student, altar server, republican and loyal friend lives in Tradinveen, Co. Kerry. His parents, Jack and Jill Kyle run a pub and grocery shop. Jack is a community leader, a problem solver, Chairman of Rockfield GAA Club, Roman Catholic and IRA Official. Jack and Jill have four children – Mary, Barry, Mark and Paul, an orphan adopted from the 'The Industrial.' Barry's best friend John is a homosexual.

Barry attends the Mercy Primary School from 1954 to 1958. His friendship with Brother Ambrose, gifted teacher and skilful Gaelic football coach, develops at 'The Small Mon' from '58 to '63. Barry transfers to 'The Big Mon' in 1963 where he encounters the traditional Brother Thomas, who is determined to win The Moran Cup. Barry suffers ongoing bullying from Bobby Collins, Vice-Principal, Free Stater and bitter enemy of the republican Kyle family since the Irish Civil War.

The Christian Brothers have high academic expectations of Barry. They are keen for Barry to become a Christian Brother. The Dominican's expect Barry to follow in the footsteps of his great-uncle Fr. Don Kyle OP while Fr. O Brien PP wants Barry to transfer to the Diocesan Seminary, 'The Dice' in Killamney. The Big Mon and The Dice are bitter rivals.

Meanwhile, Brother Ambrose, who has set up a very progressive juvenile football structure in Rockfield GAA Club, is a positive constant in Barry's adolescent life and stands up to be counted when John's homosexuality is exposed.

Many of the contemporary issues of the period – brutality, corporal punishment, Catholicism, The Irish Language, republicanism, homosexuality, adoption, The Industrial School, bullying, murder, assassination, GAA, IRA, post-Civil War tension, etc are seamlessly embroidered into this compelling story.

The story follows Barry's adolescent conflict between his religious vocation and his developing sexuality. It draws in many of the seminal events and personalities of the period – John Fitzgerald Kennedy, Martin Luther King, Jack Lynch, Donogh O Malley, the permissive '60's, Hippies, Flower Power generation, etc.

This is the first book in the enthralling Barry Kyle trilogy. It captures the ambiguity, bigotry and hypocrisy of a time, when Barry's brother, Paul is called 'a bastard from The Industrial' and his best friend John is called 'a fucking pervert.'

AVAILABLE FOR PURCHASE ONLINE
at
www.amazon.co.uk

Printed in Great Britain
by Amazon